Over-the-Counter
DRUGS

Over-the-Counter
DRUGS

Reader's Digest Association, Inc.
Pleasantville, New York / Montreal

Reader's Digest Project Staff

Senior Editor
Marianne Wait

Senior Designer
Judith Carmel

Production Technology Manager
Douglas A. Croll

Contributing Editor
Susan Carleton

Reader's Digest Health Publishing

Editorial Director
Christopher Cavanaugh

Art Director
Joan Mazzeo

Marketing Director
James H. Malloy

Vice President and General Manager
Shirrel Rhoades

The Reader's Digest Association, Inc.

Editor-in-Chief
Eric W. Schrier

President, North American Books and Home Entertainment
Thomas D. Gardner

Reader's Digest Book Produced by Rebus, Inc.

Publisher
Rodney Friedman

Editorial Director
Evan Hansen

Senior Editor
Sandra Wilmot

Contributing Editor
Marya Dalrymple

Consulting Editors
Jeremy D. Birch, Andrea Peirce, Carol Weeg

Chief of Information Resources
Tom Damrauer

Production Database Manager
John Vasiliadis

Art Director
Timothy Jeffs

Art Associate
Bree Rock

Address any comments about Guide to Drugs and Supplements: Over-the-Counter Drugs to
Reader's Digest, Editorial Director, Reader's Digest Health Publishing
Reader's Digest Road
Pleasantville, NY 10570

To order additional copies of Guide to Drugs and Supplements: Over-the-Counter Drugs,
call 1-800-846-2100

Visit our website at www.rd.com

1 3 5 7 9 10 8 6 4 2

Library of Congress Cataloging-in-Publication Data

Guide to drugs and supplements : over-the-counter drugs.
    p. cm.
    Includes index.
    ISBN 0-7621-0366-3
    1. Drugs, Nonprescription–Popular works. 2. Drugs,
Nonprescription–Encyclopedias. I. Reader's Digest Association.

RM671.A1 G85 2002
615'.1–dc21

2001048891

CONTENTS

▼

HOW TO USE THIS BOOK

▼

This book presents the essential facts on many common generic and brand name drugs in use today. With all the nonprescription, over-the-counter (OTC) drugs that are now available, it's more important than ever to be well informed on the safe and proper use of medications—whether for yourself, an aging parent, or a sick child. This book will help you to do that. It presents the facts in clear, easy-to-understand language, and in a context that will help you to make the best decisions and to use your medicines in the safest and most effective way possible.

THE BOOK CONSISTS OF THREE MAIN SECTIONS:

A General Medication Overview. The introductory portion of the book contains essential information to help you use OTC medicines wisely. The advice in *Understanding Your Medications* includes valuable tips on drug safety, as well as information about traveling with medications, proper storage, and dozens of other topics.

A-to-Z Individual Drug Profiles. The core of the book is an A-to-Z resource of nearly 100 individual drug profiles, encompassing hundreds of generic and brand name medications. Here you'll find the information you need about a particular drug and its proper use, including why it's taken, how it works, dosage guidelines, precautions, side effects, what to do in the case of an overdose, and food and drug interactions. Each profile is clearly organized in a one- to two-page format for quick, easy lookup.

A Glossary and General Index. The back pages of the book contain a comprehensive *Glossary of Drug Terms* and an *Index* to help you quickly and easily find the appropriate drug profile.

Remember, you are part of a health-care team. This book will help you to become better informed about your drugs and medications. Use it to work closely with your doctor, pharmacist, and other trusted health-care professionals, to help answer any questions you may have about getting the most out of your medications, and to obtain the best possible medical care and advice.

▼ THE DRUG PROFILE

Every medication included in this book is available as an over-the-counter (OTC) drug—which means that it is obtainable without a doctor's prescription and is distributed not only at drug stores, but also at supermarkets, chain stores, and other retail outlets.

Initially, most new medications are available only by prescription and then they are sold OTC. A drug is granted OTC status by the FDA only after a panel of experts determines that it can be used safely and effectively without a doctor's supervision—even though all drugs carry at least a few risks.

Many medications continue as prescription drugs even after an OTC version becomes available. Typically, the OTC form has a different brand name, a lower dosage, and more limited uses. OTC drugs must be taken with the same caution as prescriptions. Always read the labels, which give proper dosing and list possible food or drug interactions.

Each of the medications covered in this book is given a drug profile, which contains essential facts in an easy-to-follow, standardized, one- to two-page format. The profile provides the various names and formulations for the drug, information on its proper use or uses, guidelines for taking the drug, side effects and precautions associated with the drug, any potentially dangerous interactions with food or other medicines, and any additional facts needed to manage the medication.

The individual components of each drug profile are discussed below, with a brief description of the topics that are covered under each heading. General tips and suggestions for using your medicines safely and effectively are provided here as well. You can use this overview to get acquainted with how the profiles are organized and to obtain important general advice about your medications. After consulting a specific drug profile, or whenever you begin a new course of medication, refer to this introduction to answer questions about general drug safety.

◆ Generic and Brand Names

The drug profile identifies each drug in large, bold type at the top of the page by its generic name—a unique and standardized scientific designation that is recognized worldwide. In addition, many drugs are commonly known by

 ## GENERIC VERSUS BRAND NAME: WHICH IS BETTER?

Generic drugs have become increasingly popular since the 1980s, when the generic drug approval process was expanded and safety guidelines were issued by the Food and Drug Administration (FDA). About 250 new generic drugs are approved by the FDA each year. Generics are less expensive than brand name drugs. But are they as effective?

Ongoing supervision by the FDA helps to assure that generics sold in this country *are* as safe and effective as their brand name counterparts. The FDA requires that all generic drugs be bioequivalent to their brand name counterparts—that is, they must deliver the same amount of active ingredient to the body in a similar time frame. Furthermore, they must have similar chemical stability, so that they maintain their potency under normal circumstances for an equivalent period of time.

In addition, all drugs, including generics, must meet specifications set by the U.S. Pharmacopeial Convention, a private scientific organization that sets standards for drugs and drug products in the United States. Although there are stories in the media from time to time about the sale of substandard generic drugs, such occurrences are rare. The FDA maintains strict standards and inspection practices as well as extensive testing and monitoring of all drug manufacturing processes. About 80 percent of generic drugs sold in this country are manufactured by brand name firms in state-of-the-art plants.

You and your doctor can discuss whether generic or brand name drugs are right for you. Once you have started on a new drug therapy, it's best to stick with what you've been using—be it generic or name brand—unless your doctor says it's okay to change. There are subtle variations between some generic and brand name drugs that may make one type preferable for your situation. Switching from one form to the other could, for example, slightly alter the dose that your doctor has determined to be most suitable for your needs.

TIPS FOR TAKING YOUR MEDICATIONS

TABLETS AND CAPSULES

Tablets come in many forms besides the standard round pill. Capsules and caplets (oblong-shaped tablets) are preferred by some people because they are easier to swallow than most round tablets. Chewable tablets are good for those who have trouble swallowing any type of pill; they should be chewed thoroughly to avoid stomach upset and should not be given to children younger than age 2 (who can't chew them properly).

Some people prefer crushing tablets and mixing them with juice, water, or soft foods like applesauce to make them easier to swallow. This may be okay for some drugs, but certain medications are not designed for this. Enteric-coated tablets, for example, have a protective layer that allows the pill to dissolve in the intestine rather than the stomach. Crushing the tablet could cause stomach irritation.

Similarly, pills that have a sustained-release, timed-release, or extended-release formulation are designed to disintegrate slowly within the body and should be swallowed whole. Capsules, too, are not supposed to be broken up or cut into pieces. Check with your doctor or pharmacist before crushing any pills or tablets.

Additional Tips
- To make a pill easier to swallow, it may be helpful to drink some water before taking it and a glass of water after. It's also a good idea to stand up while swallowing.

- If a pill gets stuck in your throat, try eating a soft food such as a banana. Swallowing the food may help to carry the pill down.

EYE AND EAR MEDICATIONS

Always wash your hands before and after administering eye (ophthalmic) or ear (otic) medications. In addition, be careful not to touch the tip of the dropper or applicator to any surface, including the ear canal or eye lids, to avoid contamination. Following are additional tips for applying these medications.

Using an Eyedropper
- Tilt the head back.

- Pull the lower eyelid downward using a finger or by pinching and pulling with the thumb and index finger, creating a pocket between the eye and lower lid.

- Drop the medication into this eyelid pocket. Blink to disperse.

Applying Eye Ointments
- Pull the lower eyelid downward using a finger or by pinching and pulling with the thumb and index finger to create a pocket.

- Squeeze the tube and apply a thin strip (about a third of an inch) of ointment into this eyelid pocket. Blink to disperse.

Administering Ear Drops
- Lie down or tilt the head so that the affected ear faces up.

- For adults, pull the ear lobe up and back to straighten the ear canal. For young children, pull the ear lobe down and back.

- Drop the medication into the ear canal, but don't insert the tip of the dropper any deeper than the outer ear.

- Keep the ear facing up for a few minutes so the medication can reach the bottom of the ear canal.

RECTAL SUPPOSITORIES

A rectal suppository is a relatively large, solid, cone-shaped drug preparation. Once inserted into the rectum, it melts because of body heat and the drug is released. Suppositories may be useful for very ill patients, young children, or for others who cannot take oral medications. Lubricant suppositories may also be helpful for the treatment of constipation.

Inserting a Rectal Suppository
- The suppository should not be too soft or it will be difficult to insert. If necessary, before removing the foil wrapper, run the suppository under cold water or chill it in the refrigerator for about a half hour, until it is firm.

- Wearing a latex glove, unwrap the suppository and moisten it with water. Lie on your side and gently push the suppository, rounded end first, well up into the rectum with your finger.

- In children, gently insert the suppository no more than 3 inches into the rectum.

- Lie still and try to retain the suppository for at least 20 minutes so that the drug is absorbed.

VAGINAL MEDICATIONS

Use the special applicator that comes with your medicine and follow the directions carefully. To administer the medicine, lie on your back with your knees pulled up. Insert the applicator into the vagina as far as you can without forcing it, then press the plunger to release the medicine. Withdraw the applicator; wash it with soap and warm water.

NASAL MEDICATIONS

Blow the nose gently before administering nasal medications. After use, rinse the tip of the applicator with hot water and dry with a clean tissue. To avoid spreading infection, don't share medications with others.

Administering Nose Drops

• Tilt the head back and place the recommended number of drops in each nostril.

• Keep the head back for several minutes to allow the medicine to spread through the nasal passages.

Administering Nasal Sprays

• Keep the head upright and then squeeze the bottle firmly to spray medicine into each nostril; sniff in briskly.

• Hold the breath for a few seconds, then breathe out through the mouth.

LIQUID MEDICATIONS

Several forms of liquid medication are produced, including syrups, solutions, elixirs, and suspensions. Always measure the liquid carefully. Don't use ordinary kitchen spoons to measure out a dose; instead, use the measuring device (syringe, dropper, spoon, cup) that comes with the drug or ask your pharmacist for one.

Administering a Liquid

• To avoid a possible gagging reaction, always sit up (or prop yourself up) before taking a liquid drug.

• Drop the liquid into the side of the mouth (not the back).

one or more brand names—the name that the drug manufacturer selects to market its product. For example, ibuprofen is the generic designation for a commonly used pain reliever; Motrin, Nuprin, Medipren, and Advil are four of the brand names for ibuprofen. The drug profile includes brand names that are commonly available in the United States

Generic drug names are listed alphabetically in the main portion of the book. If you know the generic name of a drug, you can use this A-to-Z resource to quickly locate the relevant information. Note that some profiles cover combinations of two or more generic drugs, formulated as a single preparation.

Also, terms such as "hydrochloride" or "sodium" are sometimes included in a generic drug's name. In many instances the modified formulation (sometimes called a "salt") is not important, because the drug will break down into a single active ingredient in the body.

The pain reliever naproxen, for example, is sold by prescription simply as naproxen. The less powerful version of the drug that has been approved for OTC use, however, is formulated as naproxen sodium. In fact, both versions of this drug act identically once their common active ingredient (naproxen) is released in the body.

In other cases, though, a chemical modification is significant. For example, magnesium citrate, magnesium oxide, and magnesium sulfate all act differently enough in the body to qualify as separate drugs, and so each one has its own drug profile.

If you know a drug by its brand name, you can find its profile quickly by consulting the book's index, which lists both generic and brand names for drugs and the appropriate page number for their profiles. Of course, due

to space constraints, not every single medication sold around the world is included in this book. What we have selected are many of the most common generic and brand name drugs used in the United States.

◆ Available Forms

Each drug profile lists the available forms of a drug—such as a tablet, capsule, liquid, or powder. Each form has certain properties that may make it preferable for your condition or that can make taking your medications easier, safer, or more effective. If you have a skin infection, for example, you may need an antibacterial skin cream; an eye or ear infection, on the other hand, may call for ophthalmic or otic drops or ointment.

A distinction is sometimes made between local and systemic drugs. Local drugs tend to exert their effects over a limited area of the body; they include topical preparations—which are applied to the skin, eyes, ears, hair, or mucous membranes—and certain types of injections into the skin, muscles, or joints.

This contrasts with systemic drugs, which are absorbed by the bloodstream and circulated widely through many of the body's organ systems. This category includes oral preparations that are taken by mouth (such as tablets, capsules, or liquids) as well as injections (such as insulin). Locally acting formulations tend to cause fewer and less serious side effects (for example, a limited skin rash) than systemic drugs, though they do sometimes cause widespread reactions.

Formulations can also affect how rapidly a drug is absorbed, how much of the drug is absorbed, or how quickly it can take effect. An injection of a medication directly into a vein

SELECTING **OVER-THE-COUNTER DRUGS**

Over-the-counter (OTC) drugs should not be taken lightly. All drugs have side effects and need to be taken as directed—whether that direction comes from your doctor, a pharmacist, or the back of the package. To help avoid mishaps, follow the steps listed below when choosing an OTC preparation.

1. Read the label. All OTC drugs sold in the United States must meet strict labeling requirements. Follow all directions carefully.

2. Check for ingredients. Many products with similar-sounding brand names actually contain different active ingredients. Non-drowsy formulas, for example, may contain different drugs than regular formulas. Be sure to check inactive ingredients too. Some products contain dyes or fillers that can cause allergic reactions. People who are allergic to aspirin, for example, will also be allergic to the dye Yellow No. 5.

3. Be aware of combination products. Many OTC products contain multiple active ingredients, some of which may not be appropriate for you. Patients with liver disease, for example, should be wary of products that contain acetaminophen, a common ingredient in many OTC preparations.

4. Protect against tampering. Learn about the product's tamper-evident features from the label, and check the package for such signs of tampering as broken seals, puncture holes, or open or damaged wrapping. Never take medicine that is discolored, has an unusual odor, or seems suspicious in some other way. Return suspicious medicine to the store manager or pharmacist.

5. Save money by buying generics. These products are as safe and effective as their brand-name counterparts and are much less costly.

6. Be cautious when shopping overseas. Many foreign countries do not have the strict guidelines required in the United States for ensuring drug quality.

7. Check the expiration date. You do not want to buy a product that will soon expire, though you can safely use some OTC drugs past their expiration date. If stored under good conditions, most OTC drugs retain 70 to 80 percent of their potency for one or two years after the expiration date, even if the package has been opened. (Prescription drugs should never be used past their expiration date.)

8. Buy the right strength. Many OTC medications are available in multiple strengths or concentrations. Check with your doctor for advice on the potency that's right for you.

9. Watch for product reformulations. Brand-name OTC drugs occasionally are reformulated with different ingredients but retain their popular name. If you regularly take a particular OTC drug, periodically check the ingredients when restocking to be sure you are getting the same medication.

10. Don't confuse products. In addition to making different products that have similar-sounding brand names, some drug manufacturers also wrap their products in similar packaging. Double check the label when you buy a product and again when you take it, to make sure you are getting the right medication.

---

takes effect nearly immediately and its use can be critical during emergency situations. At the other end of the spectrum are the so-called controlled-release, prolonged-action, sustained-release, or timed-release preparations, including specially formulated capsules or transdermal skin patches. These are made to provide slow, uniform absorption of a drug over a period of 8 hours or longer.

Enteric-coated oral preparations are designed to keep the drug from being dissolved by stomach acids,

lessening the chance of gastrointestinal side effects. Other formulations include sublingual preparations (which are placed under the tongue to dissolve), nasal and inhalant preparations (which are breathed in through the nose or mouth), rectal suppositories, and vaginal creams or suppositories.

◆*Available as Generic*
The drug profile tells you whether or not a drug is available in a generic form. A generic drug is a copycat version of a brand-name drug—it should not be con-

fused with the generic name for a drug (see page 7). All drugs have a scientific, or generic, name, but only certain drugs are available in generic versions.

Typically, a pharmaceutical company will conduct exhaustive research and testing to launch a pioneer drug, or the first version of a new drug. In return, the company usually has patents and an exclusive license to sell that new drug for a set period, normally about 20 years from the time testing begins. The drug is usually marketed under a brand name.

Once that license expires, however, other drug companies are free to make generic versions of that drug—provided the copy is as safe and effective as the original. Generic drugs are usually sold under their generic (or scientific) name, often at half the price of the brand-name version. Commonly, there are many generic versions of a popular parent drug, and generics are available for both prescription and OTC drugs.

◆ Drug Class

Each drug is classified according to its drug class—a group of drugs that have similar chemical structures or similar actions on the body. For example, a drug that reduces fever falls into the antipyretic class; one that relieves pain belongs in the analgesic class. Some drugs have multiple functions and may therefore belong to more than one drug class. In general, however, drugs with similar chemical structures have somewhat similar effects on the body.

▼ USAGE INFORMATION

◆ Why It's Taken

The specific conditions, disorders, diseases, or symptoms for which a drug is prescribed are known as its indications. All drugs—prescription and OTC—must be approved specifically for one or more indications before they are brought to market; additional indications may later be approved by the FDA after appropriate studies have been conducted.

For OTC drugs, each of the indications listed on the medication's label must be officially approved by the FDA. For this reason, you will sometimes see OTC indications referred to as "FDA approved uses" or simply "approved uses."

◆ How It Works

This section of the drug profile briefly describes how a drug acts on or within your body to achieve its desired therapeutic effect. Some drug actions are well understood. For many drugs, however, the precise mechanism of action is unknown.

▼ DOSAGE GUIDELINES

The first safety rule for any medicine—be it OTC or prescription—is to take the correct dose at the right intervals. You should take great care to precisely follow the dosage instructions printed on OTC drug labels. Never take more (or less) than the recommended dose without first consulting your doctor or your pharmacist .

◆ Range and Frequency

The drug profile lists the usual dosage ranges for each drug. You can use these figures as general guidelines, but don't be alarmed if your doctor recommends a dosage slightly above or below the range given. The correct dosage will vary from person to person and will depend on many factors, including your age, weight, state of health, kidney and liver function, and use of other medications.

All these factors can affect how much of the drug your body absorbs, how it is distributed in your body, how long it stays there, and how much is needed for a response. Sometimes if you are taking an OTC medication on your doctor's advice, he or she may tell you to raise or lower the dose that is listed on the label.

Note that drug dosages are often given in metric units of weight, such as grams (g), milligrams (mg), or micrograms (mcg). Dosages for some

drugs, including vitamins, may be given in milliequivalents (mEq), a standard chemical unit of measure. Sometimes drug dosages are allocated per pound of body weight; this is especially useful in determining the optimal dosages for young children.

◆ Onset of Effect

Many drugs exert their effects within minutes. Common analgesics such as aspirin or acetaminophen, for example, begin to relieve pain within an hour. Often, though, you must take multiple doses of a medication before levels in your body have built up sufficiently to be effective. Usually this will occur within a day or two; however, for certain drugs, it may take several weeks for the drug to exert a noticeable effect.

◆ Duration of Effect

How long a drug exerts its effects on your body depends on the individual medication. Some stay in your system for days, or even much longer; others last only a few hours. The body metabolizes different drugs at different rates. In general, the faster a drug is metabolized, the more frequently you will need to take another dose.

The drug profile indicates how long, on average, a drug may remain in your system. Various factors, which include general health, kidney or liver function, and food or drug interactions, can significantly increase or decrease a drug's duration of action.

◆ Dietary Advice

The drug profile tells you if a medication should be taken with or without food. Food can often affect how much of the drug will be absorbed into your body, and how quickly the body absorbs it.

11

Many drugs should be taken with meals, especially with foods that contain some protein and fat. Food delays the emptying of stomach contents, allowing more time for a pill or capsule to be dissolved before entering the intestines, where many drugs are absorbed. In addition, some drugs can irritate the stomach's lining if taken on an empty stomach. Taking them with food, or even a glass of milk, can help minimize the likelihood of stomach upset or other gastrointestinal disturbances. Avoid taking medicines with coffee, tea, or other hot beverages, however, because heat can inactivate or alter some medications.

Other drugs should be taken on an empty stomach—which means at least an hour before or two hours after a meal. In general, such drugs are poorly absorbed if they're taken with food. They should, however, be taken with a glass of water.

Specific foods and drinks, including alcohol, can also interact with individual drugs. These effects are discussed under "Precautions" (see page 14) and "Food Interactions" (see page 17).

◆ Storage
Requirements for storing your medicines should be clearly indicated on the label. In general, it is recommended that most medications be kept in a cool and dry place. This usually precludes the bathroom medicine cabinet, because bathrooms tend to be humid. Similarly, drugs should not be kept near a hot kitchen stove. A bedroom or kitchen closet, which tends to be cooler and drier, may be preferable.

Some liquid medicines may need to be refrigerated. Unless your doctor or pharmacist tells you otherwise, though, it is not usually necessary to refrigerate most medications.

TRAVELING **WITH YOUR MEDICATIONS**

• Make sure you bring enough medications to last your entire trip, plus an extra supply to cover unexpected travel delays. Don't pack medications in suitcases that you plan to check; the luggage might be delayed or lost.

• If you carry syringes (say, for insulin), it's wise to also carry a note from your doctor that clearly explains your health history and medication needs; in some countries, these items may otherwise be confiscated at customs.

• Keep drugs in their original, labeled containers. Pill bottles should be stuffed with cotton to prevent damage during transit; liquid medications should be stored in self-sealing plastic bags.

• Be up to date on your immunizations. You may also need additional shots or medications for travel to certain exotic locales. Consult your doctor at least 6 weeks prior to your trip about the need for any new vaccinations or drugs. You may also want to check beforehand about where to obtain emergency medical help while you're traveling. Often a consulate can provide this information.

• Be aware that a change in climate may bring on untoward drug side effects. In hot climates, for example, drugs such as antihistamines and cold preparations can decrease your ability to perspire.

• If you are crossing several time zones and are on a fixed dosage schedule, you may have to make dosing adjustments. Discuss these and any other concerns with your doctor before you depart.

It's always a good idea to store drugs in their original containers. Discard the cotton placed at the top of pill bottles; once it is touched, it can quickly become contaminated from the bacteria on your skin. If you need to use a pill organizer, check with your doctor or pharmacist to make sure that the amount of light or moisture it lets through will not adversely affect any of your particular medicines.

If young children are around the house, be sure that you store medicines in containers with childproof caps and well out of a child's reach. In addition, don't store drugs near dangerous substances that might be taken by mistake.

◆ Missed Dose
Everyone misses a dose of medication now and then. The drug profile tells you what to do when this occurs. For some drugs, the missed dose should be taken right away. For other drugs, you can modify your dosage schedule or wait until the next scheduled dose. In general, it's better not to simply double up on missed doses. In doing so you run the risk of raising the drug concentrations in your body to dangerously high levels.

Products are available that help to remind you to take your medicines on a proper schedule. These items, sometimes called compliance aids, include check-off calendars, pill containers with sections for daily doses, electronic devices that beep or ring loudly when it's time for a dose, and also computerized pill dispensers. If you need help in selecting a one of these aids, ask your doctor or your pharmacist for advice.

TRAVELER'S **MEDICAL KIT**

Wherever you plan to travel, it's a good idea to pack certain essential items. What goes into a medical travel kit will obviously depend on where you're going, how long you're staying, and the general health condition and ages of those traveling. But there are certain basic items that it's prudent for virtually any traveler to have. The list below outlines some items that might be included in a basic medical kit. Review these and decide which might be appropriate for you to bring along. It's best to be prepared so that an unexpected injury or ailment doesn't spoil a much-anticipated trip.

HEALTH CONCERN	WHAT TO PACK
Allergies and allergic reactions	An antihistamine, such as diphenhydramine hydrochloride.
Children's and infants' special needs	Syrup of ipecac and activated charcoal (antidotes for some cases of accidental poisoning); fluid replacement formula; ear drops and antibiotic creams (in case of bacterial infection). Keep any medications in childproof containers and out of reach.
Constipation	A laxative.
Colds, cough, or sinus congestion	Throat lozenges; gargle solution; cough syrup. For air travel, a decongestant, taken a half hour before takeoff and landing, can help to ease sinus and ear discomfort.
Cuts and scrapes/ skin infections	Topical antibiotic ointment, such as iodine antiseptic or bacitracin.
Diarrhea, indigestion	Bismuth subsalicylate, loperamide, antacids, and/or antigas preparations.
Eye care	Spare pair of eyeglasses and/or contact lenses along with cleaning supplies, and a copy of your lens prescription.
Fever, headache, minor aches and pains	Aspirin, acetaminophen, naproxen, or ibuprofen.
First aid supplies	Bandages, gauze, tape, scissors, tweezers, pocket knife, safety pins, alcohol wipes, fever thermometer—stored in a waterproof case. Don't forget to bring along any health insurance or Medical Alert cards.
Insects	Insect repellent containing DEET or permethrin.
Itches, bites, skin rashes	A topical corticosteroid cream, such as hydrocortisone 1%; an antihistamine.
Motion sickness	An over-the-counter antihistamine, such as dimenhydrinate or meclizine, or a prescription scopolamine skin patch.
Nasal congestion due to colds or allergies	A decongestant, such as pseudoephedrine, and/or an antihistamine.
Sprains and strains	An elastic bandage along with an anti-inflammatory pain reliever, such as aspirin or ibuprofen.
Sun protection	Sunscreen and lip balm with an SPF of 15 or higher.
Water impurities	Water-purification tablets.

◆ Stopping the Drug

For all drugs, it's important that you follow through with the recommended course of therapy. Some drugs may take a few months to produce full benefit. Others may need to be continued on a long-term basis. If you experience bothersome side effects or don't feel that a drug is having the intended effect, talk with your doctor or pharmacist, but don't change your medication schedule on your own.

◆ Prolonged Use

If you require a drug for a chronic condition, you may need to take it for extended periods, or even a lifetime. Regular checkups or periodic testing or monitoring may be required to make sure the drug is not causing any unwanted adverse effects.

▼ SIDE EFFECTS

Along with their desired therapeutic actions, drugs typically exert other effects on the body, many of which are undesirable. Such side effects can occur with virtually all over-the-counter and prescription drugs, even when they're taken properly. Keep in mind, though, that only a small percentage of patients who are taking a drug actually experience significant side effects, even the relatively common ones.

The drug profile groups the side effects as serious, common, and less common. Serious side effects are those that may be life-threatening or otherwise have a significant impact on well-being. You should seek immediate medical assistance if you experience a serious side effect from a drug. Of course, even a mild side effect can be significant if it has a negative impact on the quality of your life.

It's a good idea to call your doctor if you are concerned about any side effect, even a seemingly minor one. Write down any problems you are having with your medicine so you will remember them when you talk with your doctor or pharmacist, and don't be afraid to ask questions.

▼ PRECAUTIONS

◆ Over 60

Drugs should be used with special caution by people older than age 60. Physiologic changes brought on by aging—including diminishing kidney and liver function, an increase in the ratio of fat to muscle, and a decrease in the amount of water in body tissues—all act to concentrate drugs and prevent them from being eliminated at a normal rate. Consequently, older adults may often require lower dosages than the standard amounts usually recommended.

According to the FDA, a good percentage of hospitalizations among older adults are caused by the side effects of drugs. Drug side effects, as well as drug and food interactions and overdose, are more common in older patients, in part because older people are much more likely than younger people to be taking medications in the first place.

The problem is compounded if multiple medications are involved, particularly when drugs are prescribed by different doctors, who may not always be aware of other medications (especially OTC drugs) that their patient is taking. In addition, studies have shown that a surprisingly sizeable percentage of elderly patients are advised to take drugs that are contraindicated for those in their age group.

It's important to let all of your doctors know of any medication you are taking—whether it is an OTC or a prescription drug—and for you to know as much as possible about the drugs you are taking. As a general rule, don't attribute any changes in mood or any new or unusual reactions or physical changes simply to old age; they may actually be drug side effects or dangerous interactions.

◆ Driving and Hazardous Work

Because some medications may cause drowsiness or confusion, they should not be used when driving, working with dangerous tools or machinery, or in other situations where a lapse in concentration could cause serious injury. If a drug makes you drowsy, talk to your doctor about scheduling doses near your bedtime, or ask about other drugs that might be substituted. Always check to see if a medicine may affect alertness and concentration before driving or engaging in a potentially hazardous activity.

◆ Alcohol

Certain medications, including many OTC drugs, can be dangerous if they are taken with alcohol. It's important for you to know whether or not to avoid alcohol whenever you begin taking a new drug. Common signs of alcohol-drug interactions include excessive sleepiness, difficulty breathing, and stomach irritation. If in doubt, the best bet is to avoid the combination of alcoholic beverages and OTC or prescription medications.

◆ Pregnancy

Some drugs are known to be harmful during pregnancy and should unequivocally be avoided during that time. A few have been shown to be safe.

But for most drugs, too few studies have been conducted for researchers to know for sure if the drug is truly dangerous to the fetus.

In general, women should try to minimize the use of OTC (and also prescription) drugs during pregnancy, though certain medications, such as vitamin supplements, may well be recommended by your doctor. This precaution should extend to alcohol (present in some drug preparations), which most experts recommend avoiding. Your specific medical needs (as assessed by your doctor) will determine if a drug is absolutely necessary. Remember that the benefits of many drugs, when indicated, far outweigh the slight possible risk to mother or fetus.

◆ *Breast Feeding*
Check with your doctor before taking any OTC medicine If you are nursing. Most drugs—including vitamins and herbal supplements—pass into breast milk to some extent, though some do so more readily and in larger amounts than others. And while most medications have little or no apparent effect on the nursing infant, some have been found to be dangerous.

The drug profile indicates whether a specific drug should be avoided by nursing mothers. As with pregnancy, it's generally best to minimize the use of medications during this time. Most experts recommend avoiding or strictly limiting alcohol intake as well. For mild pain relief, ibuprofen may be preferable to aspirin or other pain relievers, although most analgesics can be used relatively safely while breast-feeding; check with your doctor about the best choice for you.

Of course, your medical condition may require you to take certain drugs

BASIC MEDICINE SAFETY TIPS

1. Follow instructions carefully. It's essential that you take the correct dose at the proper intervals, and avoid potential interactions.

2. Keep a log of your medicines and let your doctor know your drug and medical history. Make a point of reviewing all of your medications with your primary-care doctor annually, including OTC drugs you take regularly.

3. Store medicines properly, away from sunlight, heat, and humidity. The bathroom medicine cabinet, because of the humidity, is not a good location. A locked closet—away from the reach and sight of children—is ideal.

4. Be aware of expiration dates. While you should always toss out prescription medications that have expired, you can keep many OTC drugs for one to two years after the expiration date, if they have been stored properly. Check with your doctor if you're not sure.

5. Don't take medicines in the dark. You could take the wrong pill by accident. Read the label carefully each time you take a drug to be sure you are getting the right medicine.

6. Keep emergency phone numbers handy. You should have the numbers of your doctor, emergency medical services, and the nearest poison control center readily available in case a medical emergency arises.

7. Don't be afraid to ask questions. Understand your medicines as thoroughly as possible: why you are taking them, how and when they should be taken, things to look out for. People who ask questions are more satisfied with their medical care.

8. Alert your doctor to any side effects or changes in your condition. He or she may be able to adjust your dosage or give you a substitute medication.

while breast feeding. Ask your doctor to help you weigh the risks and benefits of your drug therapy. Sometimes, a drug regimen can be suspended during the nursing period, or breast feeding can be stopped temporarily if a drug is needed for only a short time. Dosing regimens can be modified, or substitute drugs used.

◆ *Infants and Children*
Children are more sensitive than adults to many medicines. If a drug is indicated for use by children, be especially attentive to adverse reactions. If you have any concerns, talk to your doctor, pediatrician, or pharmacist.

OTC drugs, like all medications, should be given judiciously to chil-

dren. To begin, thoroughly study the label of any OTC medicine you're considering for a child to make sure the drug is indeed child-safe. If the label does not have a pediatric dose listed, don't administer it to any child under age 12. OTC drugs should not be given to any child younger than age 2 without a doctor's or pharmacist's approval. Avoid combining children's OTC remedies. Many preparations contain more than one active ingredient, and giving your child two or more different remedies can more easily lead to side effects or overdose.

Important note: Aspirin and other salicylates should not be given to children under age 16 unless your doctor instructs otherwise. When used to treat chicken pox or flu, these drugs have been associated with Reye's syndrome, a rare but potentially fatal liver disorder. Use acetaminophen or ibuprofen instead.

It's also important to remember that many OTC medications contain alcohol, which can be dangerous to small children.

◆ Special Concerns

The profile also notes any additional special concerns that you should be aware of when you're taking that particular drug. One such possibility is an allergic reaction, which occurs when the body's immune system mounts a response against a specific drug. Allergic reactions can occur with virtually any drug, including OTC medications. For example some people are allergic to NSAIDs, to certain insulin preparations, and even to some antibacterial skin creams.

Common signs of an allergic drug reaction include a skin rash, hives, and itching. Severe reactions, known by the medical term anaphylaxis, can result in swelling of the face, tongue, lips, arms, or legs; swelling can also extend to the airways, making breathing difficult; this is life-threatening emergency that requires immediate medical attention.

Call the doctor if you develop any signs of an allergic reaction to the drug. Most drug allergies respond readily to treatment. Antihistamines or topical corticosteroids may be recommended for skin rashes, hives, or itching. Bronchodilators can make breathing easier. Epinephrine relieves severe reactions.

Take note of the drug that caused the reaction and let doctors, dentists, and other health-care personnel know of it in the future. You should be careful to avoid taking that drug again, since

the allergic reaction may be more serious with subsequent doses. A medical alert tag, worn as a bracelet or necklace or carried as a card, may also be helpful. The tag states the medical concern and sometimes includes a phone number that can be dialed for a detailed medical history. In addition, be sure to read OTC drug labels carefully for any ingredients that may precipitate an allergic reaction.

◆ Overdose: Symptoms and What to Do

Virtually any drug can be toxic if taken in high enough doses, but the seriousness will depend on the individual and the particular drug taken. Every profile includes a discussion of the symptoms that are typical of an overdose and what to do if one occurs.

Accidental poisonings are a particular concern for infants and children. Supplements that contain iron are a leading cause of death in young children, who cannot metabolize the mineral well. OTC diet pills, stimulants, and decongestants are also common causes of childhood poisoning. With certain drugs, even a single tablet can be life-threatening to a small child.

Store all drugs in child-resistant containers out of the reach (and sight) of children. A child-resistant container is designed so that it takes longer than 5 minutes for 80 percent of 5-year-olds to open; it is not totally child-proof!

The elderly are also at increased risk for an overdose. They are more sensitive to some drugs and are more likely to forget exactly what time they took their last dose.

DRUGS AND CHILDREN: **SPECIAL SAFETY MEASURES**

• Keep all medications (over-the-counter and prescription) out of the reach of children. Some medicines, such as iron supplements, are very toxic to youngsters.

• Use child-resistant caps, and never leave containers uncapped.

• Never give medicine to children unless it is recommended for them on the label or by a doctor.

• Check with the doctor or pharmacist before giving a child more than one medicine at a time.

• Examine dose cups carefully. Cups may be marked with various standard abbreviations. Follow label directions.

• When using a dosing syringe that has a cap, discard the cap before using the syringe.

• Never guess when converting measuring units—from teaspoons or tablespoons to ounces, for example. Consult a reliable source, such as a pharmacist.

• Don't try to remember the dose used during previous illnesses; read the label each time.

• Never use medicine for purposes not mentioned on the label, unless so directed by a doctor.

• Check with the doctor before giving a child aspirin products. Never give aspirin to a child or teenager who has or is recovering from chicken pox, flu symptoms (nausea, vomiting, or fever), or flu. Aspirin may be associated in such patients with an increased risk of Reye's syndrome, a rare but serious illness.

FDA Consumer

Most drug poisonings work fairly quickly, though some overdose effects can take weeks to appear. Signs and symptoms of an overdose vary widely and may include listlessness, confusion, breathing difficulties, rolling eyes, unusual sleepiness, or stomach upset. If a child is involved, look around for open drug containers, and check for stains around the mouth or a strange breath odor.

If you suspect an overdose, don't panic. Call your doctor or poison control center right away. Depending on the drug, an antidote such as ipecac syrup may be recommended. It's a good idea to keep a bottle of ipecac on hand (safely stored); it induces vomiting and helps rid the body of the drug.

Some experts also recommend activated charcoal (available in drugstores, usually in liquid form), which acts to absorb the poison, preventing it from spreading through the body. (Activated charcoal should not be given with ipecac syrup, since the charcoal will absorb it).

For both antidotes, the patient must be conscious. Unconscious victims need immediate professional attention. Neither antidote should be used until you have talked with a doctor or poison control center, because in some cases, ipecac or charcoal can make a patient worse.

▼ INTERACTIONS

Drugs can interact with other drugs or particular foods or be affected by certain diseases. The drug profile indicates specific interactions to watch for. The effects can range from very mild to life-threatening. People over the age of 60 are especially prone to these interactions and should exercise particular caution.

◆ *Drug Interactions*

Drug interactions occur when two or more medications react with one another, causing adverse effects. Some drugs diminish the effectiveness of others; conversely, some can bolster other medications' actions. Drug interactions may be felt almost immediately, or they can take days, weeks, or even months to develop. It's important to note that the effects of drug interactions vary from person to person. Most patients who receive drugs that could interact do not develop notable adverse effects. On the other hand, a few patients experience life-threatening reactions.

Special care should be taken by anyone who is taking multiple medications, especially if the drugs are prescribed by different doctors. In some cases, a doctor may knowingly prescribe two potentially interacting medicines after determining that the benefits they provide will sufficiently outweigh the drawbacks of a possible interaction between them.

Check with your doctor if you are concerned about possible drug interactions or if you notice unusual symptoms. Always take care with OTC drugs; they may interact with prescription drugs or with other OTC preparations. For example, don't automatically take an OTC antacid if another drug causes stomach upset, since antacids can alter the effectiveness of certain drugs. Similarly, some vitamin or mineral supplements can interact with drugs.

◆ *Food Interactions*

Certain drugs should be taken on an empty stomach, whereas others should be taken with food. For still others, it doesn't really make a great deal of difference whether you eat or don't eat when you take them. These general dietary recommendations are covered in the drug profile under "Dietary Advice" (see page 11).

Listed in this section are specific foods or drinks that can interact with a particular drug. For example, dairy products can inactivate certain drugs. Peculiar interactions have likewise been noted between certain drugs and specific foods such as grapefruit juice (but not orange juice). The list of potential food interactions is long and drug specific. Pay close attention to the food or drink interactions for your medications to help assure you're not interfering with the proper course of drug therapy.

◆ *Disease Interactions*

The final section of each drug profile details specific diseases that can have a significant impact on the effects exerted by a particular medication. Kidney or liver disease, for example, can dramatically affect drug levels in your system. Many medications, including OTC drugs, are metabolized in the liver and excreted by way of the kidneys. If either of these organs is impaired, an excess of a drug may build up in your body, potentially resulting in a severe illness.

Many other disorders, such as diabetes mellitus or heart disease, may also affect your body's response to medication—including the OTC drugs you regularly take for such unrelated conditions as allergies or headaches. It's important to tell your doctor about all diseases or conditions that you have, even if they seem to have no relevance to your immediate medical concerns.

A to Z
Drug Profiles

ACETAMINOPHEN

Available in: Capsules, caplets, tablets, powder, liquid, suppositories
Available as Generic? Yes
Drug Class: Analgesic; antipyretic (fever reducer)

▼ USAGE INFORMATION

WHY IT'S TAKEN
To treat mild to moderate pain and fever, including simple headaches, muscle aches, and mild forms of arthritis. Acetaminophen is useful for patients who cannot take aspirin, such as those taking anticoagulants or suffering from gastrointestinal ulcers or bleeding disorders.

HOW IT WORKS
Acetaminophen appears to interfere with the action of prostaglandins, substances in the body that cause inflammation and make nerves more sensitive to pain impulses. It also relieves fever, probably by acting on the heat-regulating center of the brain.

▼ DOSAGE GUIDELINES

RANGE AND FREQUENCY
For adults and teenagers: 325 to 650 mg every 4 to 6 hours, or 1 g, 3 to 4 times a day, as needed. Extended-release caplets: Take 2 every 8 hours. Maximum dosage with short-term therapy should not exceed 4 g a day; with long-term therapy it should not exceed 2.6 g a day unless otherwise prescribed by your doctor. For children 12 years and under: Consult a pediatrician for the proper dose. Liquid form may be recommended for young children.

ONSET OF EFFECT
Within 15 to 30 minutes.

DURATION OF ACTION
3 to 4 hours; 8 hours for extended-release form.

DIETARY ADVICE
Take it with water 30 minutes before or 2 hours after meals. It may be taken with milk to minimize stomach upset. If you are on a salt-restricted diet, be sure to account for the sodium present in the powder form of acetaminophen.

STORAGE
Store in a tightly sealed container away from heat and direct light. Refrigerate liquid forms (to make them more palatable) and rectal suppositories. Do not allow the medication to freeze.

MISSED DOSE
Take it as soon as you remember. If it is near the time for the next dose, skip the missed dose and resume your regular dosage schedule. Do not double the next dose.

STOPPING THE DRUG
Unless directed otherwise by your doctor, limit use to 5 days for children under 12 and 10 days for adults.

PROLONGED USE
Prolonged use may lead to liver problems, kidney problems, or anemia in some patients. Talk to your doctor about the need for periodic physical examinations and laboratory tests.

▼ PRECAUTIONS

Over 60: Adverse reactions may be more likely and more severe in older patients; lower doses may be warranted.

Driving and Hazardous Work: No problems are expected.

Alcohol: Avoid alcohol; combining the two can cause serious liver problems. Patients with a history of alcohol abuse should not use acetaminophen except under close supervision by a doctor.

Pregnancy: No problems have been reported. Consult your doctor if you are or plan to become pregnant.

Breast Feeding: No problems have been reported.

Infants and Children: No problems are expected; however, some formulations are sweetened with aspartame, which should not be consumed by children with phenylketonuria.

OVERDOSE
Symptoms: Nausea, vomiting, appetite loss, abdominal pain, excessive sweating, confusion, drowsiness or exhaustion, stomach tenderness, heartbeat irregularities, yellowing of the skin and eyes.

What to Do: If you suspect an overdose, seek medical aid immediately, even if no symptoms are present. Steps must be taken promptly to avoid potentially fatal liver damage.

▼ INTERACTIONS

DRUG INTERACTIONS
Consult your doctor for specific advice if you are taking anticoagulants (such as warfarin), aspirin, an NSAID, barbiturates, carbamazepine, hydantoins, rifampin, sulfinpyrazone, isoniazid, nicotine, or zidovudine.

FOOD INTERACTIONS
No known food interactions.

DISEASE INTERACTIONS
Consult your doctor before taking this drug if you have liver or kidney disease, diabetes mellitus, phenylketonuria, or a history of alcohol abuse.

⬇ SIDE EFFECTS ⬇

SERIOUS
Allergic reaction causing rash, itching, hives, swelling, or breathing difficulty; yellow-tinged skin and eyes (indicating liver damage). Seek medical assistance immediately.

COMMON
No common side effects have been reported.

LESS COMMON
Sore throat and fever (not present before treatment and not caused by the condition being treated), extreme fatigue or weakness, unexplained bleeding or bruising, blood in urine, painful, decreased, or frequent urination.

ACETAMINOPHEN/ASPIRIN/CAFFEINE

Available in: Tablets, caplets, oral powder
Available as Generic? No
Drug Class: Analgesic

▼ USAGE INFORMATION

WHY IT'S TAKEN
For the temporary relief of mild to moderate pain associated with arthritis or migraines.

HOW IT WORKS
Acetaminophen and aspirin both appear to interfere with the production of prostaglandins, naturally occurring substances in the body that cause inflammation and make nerves more sensitive to pain impulses. Caffeine is believed to enhance the effectiveness of pain relievers.

▼ DOSAGE GUIDELINES

RANGE AND FREQUENCY
Because the amount of each of the components varies with different brands, consult your doctor for the appropriate dose. The following are general guidelines. Adults and teenagers—Tablets and caplets: 1 to 2 pills every 3 to 6 hours, as needed and depending on the strength of the product. Do not take more than 8 pills in a 24-hour period. Oral powder: 1 packet followed immediately by a full glass of water every 6 hours. Children—Generally not recommended for children.

ONSET OF EFFECT
Unknown.

DURATION OF ACTION
Unknown.

DIETARY ADVICE
Should be taken with food or a full glass of water to minimize stomach upset.

STORAGE
Store in a tightly sealed container protected from heat, moisture, and direct light.

MISSED DOSE
Skip the missed dose and then resume your regular dosage schedule. Do not double the next dose.

STOPPING THE DRUG
You may stop taking the drug whenever you choose.

PROLONGED USE
This combination is indicated for short-term use only. Side effects are more likely with prolonged use.

▼ PRECAUTIONS

Over 60: Adverse reactions may be more common and more severe.

Driving and Hazardous Work: May cause drowsiness or vision difficulties.

Alcohol: Do not consume more than 2 alcohol-containing beverages a day.

Pregnancy: Discuss with your doctor the relative risks and benefits of using this drug while pregnant. This drug should not be used during the last 3 months of pregnancy.

Breast Feeding: This drug may pass into breast milk; consult your doctor for specific advice.

Infants and Children: Consult your pediatrician. This drug is not recommended for children under 16, since the aspirin component may cause a rare but life-threatening liver condition known as Reye's syndrome.

Special Concerns: Be sure your doctor knows you are taking this medication; it can interfere with the results of some blood and urine tests. Patients allergic to aspirin should not take this drug.

OVERDOSE
Symptoms: Nausea and vomiting, disorientation, seizures, rapid breathing, ringing or buzzing in the ears, fever, appetite loss, abdominal pain, excessive sweating, drowsiness or exhaustion, stomach tenderness, heartbeat irregularities, yellow discoloration of the skin and eyes, agitation, anxiety, restlessness, delirium.

What to Do: Call your doctor, emergency medical services (EMS), or the nearest poison control center immediately.

▼ INTERACTIONS

DRUG INTERACTIONS
Consult your doctor before taking this drug if you are currently taking any of the following: blood pressure medication, gout or arthritis drugs, anticoagulants such as warfarin, antidiabetic agents, steroids, seizure medication, NSAIDs, barbiturates, nicotine, zidovudine (AZT), isoniazid, a central nervous system stimulant, a monoamine oxidase (MAO) inhibitor, amantadine, OTC cold and allergy medications, or asthma medicine.

FOOD INTERACTIONS
Do not drink large amounts of caffeine-containing beverages like coffee, tea, cola, cocoa, or chocolate milk.

DISEASE INTERACTIONS
Consult your doctor if you have liver or kidney disease, diabetes mellitus, phenylketonuria, a history of alcohol abuse, asthma, a bleeding disorder, congestive heart failure, gout, high blood pressure, thyroid disease, a peptic ulcer, anxiety, panic attacks, agoraphobia, or insomnia.

≣ SIDE EFFECTS ≣

SERIOUS
Difficulty swallowing; dizziness, lightheadedness, or fainting; flushing, redness, or change in color of skin; difficulty breathing, shortness of breath, tightness in the chest, or wheezing; sudden decrease in urine output; swelling of face, eyelids, or lips; black or tarry stools; unusual bleeding or bruising; yellow discoloration of the skin and eyes (indicating liver damage). Call your doctor immediately.

COMMON
Indigestion, nausea and vomiting, stomach pain.

LESS COMMON
Sleeping difficulty, nervousness, irritability.

ALUMINUM SALTS

Available in: Tablets, capsules, oral suspension, gel
Available as Generic? Yes
Drug Class: Antacid

▼ USAGE INFORMATION

WHY IT'S TAKEN
To treat heartburn, acid indigestion, sour stomach, peptic ulcers, gastritis, esophagitis, and gastroesophageal reflux. May also be used to treat or prevent excess phosphate in the blood or to prevent urinary phosphate stones.

HOW IT WORKS
Aluminum salts neutralize stomach acid and reduce the action of pepsin, a digestive enzyme. This provides symptomatic relief from excess stomach acid.

▼ DOSAGE GUIDELINES

RANGE AND FREQUENCY
1 to 2 tablets or capsules or 5 to 30 ml suspension or gel as often as every 2 hours, up to 12 times per day. Take the dose between meals unless your doctor directs otherwise. When used as sole treatment of peptic ulcer or esophagitis, take it 1 and 3 hours after meals and at bedtime. Tablets should be chewed.

ONSET OF EFFECT
Within minutes.

DURATION OF ACTION
20 minutes to 3 hours.

DIETARY ADVICE
Avoid a low-phosphate diet during prolonged use, unless your doctor directs otherwise. Some recommended high-phosphate foods include red meat, poultry, fish, eggs, dark green leafy vegetables, dairy products, and nuts.

STORAGE
Store in a tightly sealed container and protect from heat, moisture, and direct light. Refrigerate liquid forms.

MISSED DOSE
Take it as soon as you remember. Do not double the next dose.

STOPPING THE DRUG
Take as directed.

PROLONGED USE
Do not take it for more than 2 weeks unless your doctor recommends otherwise.

▼ PRECAUTIONS

Over 60: Constipation or intestinal trouble is more common in older persons. Older patients who have or who are at high risk for osteoporosis or other bone disorders should avoid frequent use of this medicine.

Driving and Hazardous Work: No special precautions are necessary.

Alcohol: Alcohol decreases the effect of antacids.

Pregnancy: Consult your doctor before taking aluminum salts while pregnant.

Breast Feeding: Aluminum-containing antacids pass into breast milk. It is unknown whether this poses any risk to nursing infants. Consult your doctor for advice.

Infants and Children: Antacids should not be dispensed to children under age 6 unless otherwise instructed by a physician.

Special Concerns: Use over-the-counter antacids only occasionally unless otherwise directed by your doctor. Persistent heartburn that is not readily relieved by antacids may be a signal of a heart attack or another serious disorder. In such cases, seek medical help promptly.

OVERDOSE
Symptoms: Shallow breathing, dry mouth, constipation or diarrhea, confusion, headache, weakness or fatigue, bone pain, stupor.

What to Do: Seek medical assistance immediately.

▼ INTERACTIONS

DRUG INTERACTIONS
Other medications may lose their effectiveness when taken within 1 hour of antacids. Consult your doctor for specific advice if you are taking amphetamines, bisacodyl, citrates, chenodiol, digoxin, enteric coated medications, iron salts, isoniazid, ketoconazole, mecamylamine, methenamine, penicillamine, phosphates, nitrofurantoin, quinidine, salicylates, or tetracyclines.

FOOD INTERACTIONS
Taking an aluminum salt with food can decrease its activity. Wait at least 60 minutes after eating before taking it.

DISEASE INTERACTIONS
Do not take aluminum salts if you have any symptoms of appendicitis or an inflamed bowel (abdominal pain, cramps, soreness, bloating, nausea, vomiting). Aluminum salts are not recommended for Alzheimer's patients. Consult your doctor if you have chronic constipation, colitis, ileostomy, colostomy, intestinal or stomach blockage, bone fractures, diarrhea, kidney disease, hypophosphatemia, heart disease, liver disease, edema, stomach bleeding, intestinal bleeding.

≡ SIDE EFFECTS ≡

SERIOUS
Severe and continuing constipation, dizziness, lightheadedness, and heartbeat irregularities. Bone loss may occur, especially with prolonged use in dialysis patients. Hypophosphatemia (too little phosphate in the blood) may occur with prolonged use and a low-phosphate diet; symptoms include bone pain, fractures, muscle weakness, loss of appetite, mood changes, a general feeling of discomfort, swelling of the wrists and ankles, unusual weight loss, and anemia (decreased number of red blood cells; symptoms include weakness and fatigue).

COMMON
Chalky taste.

LESS COMMON
Mild constipation, stomach cramps, speckling or whitish coloration of stools, increased thirst, nausea and vomiting.

ASPIRIN

Available in: Tablets, capsules
Available as Generic? Yes
Drug Class: Nonsteroidal anti-inflammatory drug (NSAID); analgesic; anticoagulant

▼ USAGE INFORMATION

WHY IT'S TAKEN
For mild to moderate everyday pain and inflammation; to reduce fever; to prevent the formation of blood clots, a primary cause of heart attack, stroke, and other circulatory problems; to ease the joint inflammation, pain, and stiffness of arthritis.

HOW IT WORKS
Nonsteroidal anti-inflammatory drugs (NSAIDs) such as aspirin inhibit the release of chemicals in the body called prostaglandins, which play a role in inflammation, though it is unknown exactly how they exert their pain-relieving, fever-reducing, and anti-inflammatory effects.

▼ DOSAGE GUIDELINES

RANGE AND FREQUENCY
For pain or fever: 325 to 650 mg every 4 hours as needed. For prevention of blood clots: 80 to 100 mg daily or every other day. For arthritis: 3,600 to 5,400 mg daily in 2 or more divided doses.

ONSET OF EFFECT
30 minutes.

DURATION OF ACTION
For pain relief, up to 4 hours.

DIETARY ADVICE
Swallow aspirin with food or a full glass of water to lessen stomach irritation.

STORAGE
Store in a tightly sealed container away from heat and direct light.

MISSED DOSE
For pain and fever, take a missed dose as soon as you remember, then wait 4 hours for your next dose. For arthritis, take the aspirin as soon as you remember up to 2 hours late, then return to your regular schedule.

STOPPING THE DRUG
For pain and fever, stop when relief is achieved. For arthritis and blood clotting, consult your doctor about stopping.

PROLONGED USE
Talk to your doctor about the need for medical examinations or laboratory tests if you must take aspirin regularly for a prolonged period.

▼ PRECAUTIONS

Over 60: Gastrointestinal bleeding and irritation are more likely to occur in older persons taking this drug.

Driving and Hazardous Work: The use of aspirin should not impair your ability to perform such tasks safely.

Alcohol: Alcohol intake should be limited because it increases the risk of stomach irritation and bleeding.

Pregnancy: Do not use aspirin during the last 3 months of pregnancy unless prescribed by your doctor.

Breast Feeding: Aspirin passes into breast milk. Avoid it or do not nurse.

Infants and Children: Do not give aspirin to children under age 16 unless your doctor instructs otherwise, since it may cause a very rare but life-threatening condition known as Reye's syndrome.

OVERDOSE
Symptoms: Nausea, disorientation, seizures, vomiting, rapid breathing, fever.

What to Do: Call your doctor, emergency medical services (EMS), or the nearest poison control center immediately.

▼ INTERACTIONS

DRUG INTERACTIONS
Consult your doctor before taking aspirin if you currently take a blood pressure medication, a medication for gout, an arthritis drug, an anticoagulant such as warfarin, a diabetes medication, a steroid, or an antiseizure medication.

FOOD INTERACTIONS
No known adverse food interactions. Taking aspirin with caffeine-containing foods or beverages may actually enhance the medicine's pain-relieving effects.

DISEASE INTERACTIONS
Consult your doctor about taking aspirin if you have asthma, a bleeding disorder, congestive heart failure, diabetes mellitus, gout, hemophilia, high blood pressure, kidney disease, liver disease, thyroid disease, or a peptic ulcer.

≡ SIDE EFFECTS ≡

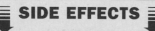

SERIOUS
Vomiting, agitation, extreme fatigue, confusion; allergic reaction causing troubled breathing, redness of face, itching, swelling of face, lips, or eyelids. These are symptoms of Reye's syndrome, a rare but serious disorder that is most likely to affect patients under the age of 16. Seek emergency medical attention immediately.

COMMON
Stomach upset, rash, nausea, ringing in the ears.

LESS COMMON
Insomnia.

ASPIRIN/CAFFEINE

Available in: Tablets
Available as Generic? No
Drug Class: Nonsteroidal anti-inflammatory drug (NSAID); analgesic; antirheumatic

▼ USAGE INFORMATION

WHY IT'S TAKEN
For mild to moderate every-day pain and inflammation; to reduce fever; to ease the joint inflammation, pain, and stiffness associated with arthritis.

HOW IT WORKS
Aspirin appears to interfere with the production of prostaglandins, naturally occurring substances in the body that cause inflammation and make nerves more sensitive to pain impulses. Caffeine may enhance the effectiveness of pain relievers.

▼ DOSAGE GUIDELINES

RANGE AND FREQUENCY
Adults—For pain or fever: 325 to 650 mg every 4 hours as needed. For arthritis: 3,600 to 5,400 mg daily in divided doses. Children 9 years of age and older under a doctor's supervision—For arthritis: 80 to 100 mg per 2.2 lbs (1 kg) of body weight a day in divided doses.

ONSET OF EFFECT
For pain, inflammation, or fever: within 30 minutes. For arthritis: may take 2 to 3 weeks of treatment to achieve maximum effect.

DURATION OF ACTION
For pain relief, up to 4 hours.

DIETARY ADVICE
Take with food or a full glass of water to lessen risk of stomach irritation.

STORAGE
Store in a tightly sealed container protected from heat, moisture, and direct light.

MISSED DOSE
For pain and fever, take a missed dose as soon as you remember, then wait 4 hours for your next dose. For arthritis, take as soon as you remember up to 2 hours late, then return to your regular dosing schedule.

STOPPING THE DRUG
For pain and fever, stop when relief is achieved. For arthritis, consult your doctor about stopping therapy.

PROLONGED USE
Talk to your doctor about the need for regular medical examinations or laboratory tests if you must take this medication regularly for a prolonged period.

▼ PRECAUTIONS

Over 60: Gastrointestinal bleeding and irritation are more likely to occur in older persons taking aspirin.

Driving and Hazardous Work: No special precautions are necessary.

Alcohol: Alcohol intake should be limited because it increases the risk of stomach irritation and bleeding.

Pregnancy: Do not use this drug during the last 3 months of pregnancy unless prescribed by your doctor.

Breast Feeding: Aspirin passes into breast milk. Avoid it or do not nurse.

Infants and Children: Do not give aspirin-containing products to children under age 16 unless your doctor instructs you to do otherwise because it may cause a very rare but life-threatening condition known as Reye's syndrome.

OVERDOSE
Symptoms: Nausea, disorientation, seizures, vomiting, rapid breathing, fever.

What to Do: Call your doctor or contact the nearest emergency medical services (EMS) or poison control center immediately.

▼ INTERACTIONS

DRUG INTERACTIONS
Consult your doctor before taking this drug if you currently take a blood pressure medication, a medication for gout, an arthritis drug, an anticoagulant such as warfarin, a diabetes medication, a steroid, or medication to control seizures.

FOOD INTERACTIONS
No known interactions.

DISEASE INTERACTIONS
Consult your doctor about taking this drug if you have asthma, a bleeding disorder, congestive heart failure, diabetes mellitus, gout, hemophilia, high blood pressure, kidney disease, liver disease, thyroid disease, or a peptic ulcer.

≡ SIDE EFFECTS ≡

SERIOUS
Vomiting, agitation, extreme fatigue, confusion; allergic reaction causing troubled breathing, redness of face, itching, swelling of face, lips, or eyelids. These are symptoms of Reye's syndrome, a rare but serious disorder that is most likely to affect patients under the age of 16. Seek emergency medical attention immediately.

COMMON
Stomach upset, rash, nausea, ringing in the ears.

LESS COMMON
Insomnia.

ATTAPULGITE

Available in: Oral suspension, tablets, chewable tablets
Available as Generic? Yes
Drug Class: Antidiarrheal

▼ USAGE INFORMATION

WHY IT'S TAKEN
To treat diarrhea.

HOW IT WORKS
Attapulgite is believed to bind to and remove large volumes of bacteria and toxins from the digestive tract. It may also reduce the fluidity of the stool associated with diarrhea. There is some debate regarding attapulgite's effectiveness.

▼ DOSAGE GUIDELINES

RANGE AND FREQUENCY
Adults and teenagers—Suspension and tablets: 1,200 to 1,500 mg taken after each loose bowel movement; take no more than 9,000 mg in 24 hours. Chewable tablets: 1,200 mg after each loose bowel movement; take no more than 8,400 mg in 24 hours. Children ages 6 to 12—Suspension and chewable tablets: 600 mg after each loose bowel movement; take no more than 4,200 mg in 24 hours. Tablets: 750 mg after each loose bowel movement; take no more than 4,500 mg in 24 hours. Children ages 3 to 6–Suspension and chewable tablets: 300 mg after each loose bowel movement; take no more than 2,100 mg in 24 hours. Tablets: Should not be taken by children in this age group.

ONSET OF EFFECT
Unknown.

DURATION OF ACTION
Unknown.

DIETARY ADVICE
A mild diet is recommended when recovering from diarrhea. Bananas, rice, applesauce, and plain toast are good choices. Be sure to get plenty of fluids.

STORAGE
Store in a tightly sealed container and protect from heat, moisture, and direct light.

MISSED DOSE
Take it as soon as you remember. However, if it is near the time for the next dose, skip the missed dose and resume your regular dosage schedule. Do not double the next dose.

STOPPING THE DRUG
You may stop taking the drug if you feel better before the scheduled end of therapy.

PROLONGED USE
If diarrhea has not improved or has gotten worse in 2 days, or if you develop a fever, call your doctor.

▼ PRECAUTIONS

Over 60: Older persons with diarrhea are more likely to experience excessive loss of body fluid and therefore are advised to increase their fluid intake accordingly.

Driving and Hazardous Work: The use of attapulgite should not impair your ability to perform such tasks safely.

Alcohol: Avoid alcohol.

Pregnancy: Attapulgite is not absorbed by the body and is not expected to cause problems during pregnancy.

Breast Feeding: Attapulgite is not absorbed by the body and is not expected to cause problems while nursing.

Infants and Children: Should not be given to children under the age of 3 without consulting your doctor. Be sure your child drinks a sufficient amount of fluids.

Special Concerns: In addition to taking attapulgite, it is important to replace the body fluids lost because of diarrhea. During the first day you should drink ample amounts of clear liquids, such as decaffeinated colas, ginger ale, and decaffeinated tea, and eat gelatin. On the following day you should continue your fluid intake and eat bland foods, such as applesauce, cooked cereals, and bread. Do not take attapulgite if your diarrhea is accompanied by blood or mucus in the stools.

OVERDOSE
Symptoms: No cases of overdose have been reported.

What to Do: An overdose is unlikely to be life-threatening. However, if someone takes a much larger dose than prescribed, seek medical assistance immediately.

▼ INTERACTIONS

DRUG INTERACTIONS
Other drugs may interact with attapulgite. If you are taking any other medication, do not take it within 2 to 3 hours before or after taking a dose of attapulgite.

FOOD INTERACTIONS
Eating fried or spicy foods, bran, fruits, vegetables, or drinking caffeinated or alcoholic beverages can make diarrhea worse.

DISEASE INTERACTIONS
Consult your doctor if you have an intestinal illness or any other medical condition.

≡ SIDE EFFECTS ≡

SERIOUS
No serious side effects are associated with attapulgite. However, loss of body water due to diarrhea can cause dry mouth, increased thirst, dizziness, lightheadedness, decreased urination, and wrinkling of skin. Call your doctor immediately if these symptoms develop.

COMMON
Constipation.

LESS COMMON
There are no less-common side effects associated with the use of attapulgite.

BACITRACIN

Available in: Ophthalmic ointment and solution; dermatologic (skin) ointment
Available as Generic? Yes
Drug Class: Antibiotic

▼ USAGE INFORMATION

WHY IT'S TAKEN
Dermatologic (skin) ointment is available over the counter for application to minor cuts and abrasions to prevent infection. Ophthalmic preparations are prescribed by a doctor for application to the eyelids or into the eye to treat early minor bacterial infections of the eyelids or conjunctiva (the mucous membranes that line the inner surface of the eyelids).

HOW IT WORKS
Hinders the ability of bacteria to manufacture cell walls, which causes cell death.

▼ DOSAGE GUIDELINES

RANGE AND FREQUENCY
Dermatologic ointment: Apply to a small cut or abrasion 2 times daily. Ophthalmic preparations: Apply to the eye 1 or more times daily.

ONSET OF EFFECT
Unknown.

DURATION OF ACTION
Unknown.

DIETARY ADVICE
No special restrictions.

STORAGE
Store in a tightly sealed container away from heat and direct light.

MISSED DOSE
Apply it as soon as you remember and resume your regular dosage schedule.

STOPPING THE DRUG
You can stop using the dermatologic ointment as soon as the cut or abrasion is sufficiently healed. The decision to stop using the ophthalmic preparation should be made by your doctor.

PROLONGED USE
Ongoing observation is needed when the ointment is used, to detect any possible overgrowth of bacterial organisms that are not susceptible to the drug (a complication known as superinfection).

▼ PRECAUTIONS

Over 60: No special problems are expected.

Driving and Hazardous Work: Ophthalmic ointment may cloud vision; caution is advised during use.

Alcohol: No special precautions required.

Pregnancy: Before using bacitracin, tell your doctor if you are pregnant or plan to become pregnant.

Breast Feeding: Bacitracin may pass into breast milk. Consult your doctor for specific advice.

Infants and Children: No special problems are expected in this group.

Special Concerns: Bacitracin preparations should not be used if you have a history of sensitivity or allergy to bacitracin or any of the other components in the ointment.

OVERDOSE
Symptoms: Severe eye pain, headache, rapid change in vision, sudden appearance of floating spots, acute redness of eye, pain on exposure to light, double vision, itching, burning, inflammation.

What to Do: Call your doctor, emergency medical services (EMS), or the nearest poison control center immediately.

▼ INTERACTIONS

DRUG INTERACTIONS
No other drugs should be applied topically when using bacitracin unless otherwise instructed by your doctor. Bacitracin has not been shown to have any significant interactions with medications taken orally.

FOOD INTERACTIONS
No known food interactions.

DISEASE INTERACTIONS
Caution is advised when using bacitracin. Consult your doctor so other appropriate treatment can be started immediately if superinfection (see Prolonged Use) with nonsusceptible bacteria occurs during therapy.

≡ SIDE EFFECTS ≡

SERIOUS
Dermatologic and ophthalmic ointment: Rare severe allergic reaction that may cause hives, breathing difficulty, or at the extreme, total closure of the airways with potentially fatal anaphylactic shock. Contact emergency medical services (EMS) immediately. Ophthalmic preparations only: Severe eye pain, headache, rapid change in vision, sudden appearance of floating spots, acute redness of eye, pain on exposure to light, double vision, itching, burning, inflammation. Call your doctor or ophthalmologist immediately.

COMMON
No common side effects have been reported.

LESS COMMON
Dermatologic ointment: Irritation or skin allergy at the site of application, marked by redness, burning, itching, or the development of a rash.

BENZOCAINE

Available in: Cream, ointment, aerosol spray, dental paste, lozenges, solution
Available as Generic? No
Drug Class: Anesthetic

▼ USAGE INFORMATION

WHY IT'S TAKEN
To relieve minor pain and itching of the skin caused by mild burns, bites, cuts, abrasions, and contact dermatitis (skin inflammation caused by contact with an irritant such as poison ivy, or by an allergic response to certain metals or other substances). Dental forms of benzocaine are used to treat pain caused by toothache, teething, cold sores, canker sores, dentures, or other dental appliances.

HOW IT WORKS
Benzocaine interferes with the ability of certain nerves to conduct electrical signals, which blocks the transmission of nerve impulses that carry pain messages.

▼ DOSAGE GUIDELINES

RANGE AND FREQUENCY
Skin cream, ointment, aerosol spray: Apply to affected area 3 or 4 times a day as needed. Dental paste: Apply as needed. Lozenges: 1 lozenge dissolved in the mouth every 2 hours as needed. Aerosol dental solution: 1 or 2 sprays of at least 1 second each, taken as needed.

ONSET OF EFFECT
Within minutes.

DURATION OF ACTION
Unknown.

DIETARY ADVICE
Forms applied to skin: Can be taken without regard to diet. Oral and dental forms: Do not eat or drink anything for 1 hour after using medicine.

STORAGE
Store in a tightly sealed container away from heat and direct light.

MISSED DOSE
Take it as soon as you remember. If it is near the time for the next dose, skip the missed dose and resume your regular dosage schedule. Do not double the next dose.

STOPPING THE DRUG
It is advisable to take the medication as prescribed for the full treatment period. However, you may stop taking the drug before the scheduled end of therapy if you are feeling better.

PROLONGED USE
For skin pain or discomfort: Check with your doctor if the condition does not improve within 7 days. For dental pain: If used temporarily for a toothache, arrange for proper dental treatment as soon as possible. For sore throat: Check with your doctor if pain lasts more than 2 days.

▼ PRECAUTIONS

Over 60: Skin: No information is available. Dental use: Adverse reactions may be more likely and more severe in older patients.

Driving and Hazardous Work: No special warnings.

Alcohol: No special precautions are necessary.

Pregnancy: Benzocaine has not been reported to cause problems in pregnancy.

Breast Feeding: No problems are expected.

Infants and Children: Dental paste can be used in teething babies 4 months and older. Use of other forms of benzocaine is not recommended for children under 2 unless prescribed by your doctor.

Special Concerns: Do not swallow the dental form unless your doctor has instructed you to do so.

OVERDOSE
Symptoms: Both skin and dental forms: Blurred or double vision; confusion; convulsions; dizziness or lightheadedness; drowsiness; feeling hot, cold, or numb; headache; increased sweating; ringing or buzzing in ears; shivering or trembling; slow or irregular heartbeat; trouble breathing; anxiety, nervousness, or restlessness; pale skin; unusual fatigue.

What to Do: Call your doctor, emergency medical services (EMS), or the nearest poison control center immediately.

▼ INTERACTIONS

DRUG INTERACTIONS
With dental benzocaine, consult your doctor for specific advice if you are taking cholinesterase inhibitors or sulfonamides.

FOOD INTERACTIONS
No known food interactions.

DISEASE INTERACTIONS
Consult your doctor if you have any other condition affecting the mouth or skin.

≡ SIDE EFFECTS ≡

SERIOUS
Skin: Severe allergic reaction, producing large, red, hive-like swellings on the skin. Dental use: Large swellings in the mouth or throat. Call your doctor immediately.

COMMON
No common side effects are associated with the skin product or the dental product.

LESS COMMON
Contact dermatitis (skin irritation), causing mild burning, stinging, swelling, itching, redness, or tenderness not present before treatment; hives in or around the mouth.

BENZOYL PEROXIDE

Available in: Lotion, cream, gel, pads, cleansing bar, facial mask, stick
Available as Generic? Yes
Drug Class: Acne drug

▼ USAGE INFORMATION

WHY IT'S TAKEN
To treat mild to moderate acne. In more severe cases benzoyl peroxide may be used in conjunction with other acne treatments, such as antibiotics, retinoic acid preparations, and sulfur- or salicylic-acid-containing medications. It may also be used to treat pressure sores and other skin disorders.

HOW IT WORKS
Benzoyl peroxide slowly releases oxygen, which has an antibacterial effect (bacteria are a primary cause of acne). It also causes peeling and drying of skin, which helps to eliminate blackheads and whiteheads.

▼ DOSAGE GUIDELINES

RANGE AND FREQUENCY
For the cream, gel, lotion, or stick form of benzoyl, first wash the affected area of skin with medicated soap and water. Pat dry gently with a towel; apply enough medicine to cover the affected area and rub in gently once or twice a day. For the shave cream form, wet the area to be shaved, apply a small amount of the cream, rub over the entire area, shave, then rinse the area and pat it dry. Check with your doctor about using aftershave lotions. If you have a fair complexion, start with a single daily application at bedtime. Keep the medicine away from eyes, nose, and mouth.

ONSET OF EFFECT
1 to several weeks.

DURATION OF ACTION
Up to 24 hours.

DIETARY ADVICE
This medication may be used without regard to diet.

STORAGE
Store in a tightly sealed container away from heat and direct light.

MISSED DOSE
If you miss a scheduled application, apply it as soon as you remember and then resume regular use.

≡ SIDE EFFECTS ≡

SERIOUS
Allergic reaction causing burning, blistering, crusting, itching, severe redness, and swelling of skin. Contact your doctor right away.

COMMON
Mild dryness and peeling of skin.

LESS COMMON
Excessive dryness, unusual feeling of warmth or heat, mild stinging, redness, irritation. This medicine may cause a rash or intensify sunburn in areas of the skin exposed to sunlight or ultraviolet light; avoid excessive sun exposure and tell your doctor if a skin reaction occurs.

STOPPING THE DRUG
Although benzoyl peroxide can be discontinued when acne improves, stopping usually leads to a recurrence of acne.

PROLONGED USE
Check with your doctor if you do not see improvement within 4 to 6 weeks. Other medications may be necessary to control acne and to prevent permanent scarring.

▼ PRECAUTIONS

Over 60: No special problems are expected.

Driving and Hazardous Work: No special warnings.

Alcohol: No special warnings.

Pregnancy: Problems in pregnancy have not been documented, but the manufacturer recommends that the medicine should not be used by pregnant women unless it is considered essential.

Breast Feeding: Benzoyl peroxide may pass into breast milk. Ask your doctor about its use during breast feeding.

Infants and Children: Studies on this medicine have been done only with teenagers and adults, so there is no specific information about its use with other age groups. Nonetheless, no special side effects or problems are expected in children over 12. No studies have been done in children under 12. Use and dose must be determined by a doctor.

OVERDOSE
Symptoms: Overapplication to the skin may cause burning, itching, scaling, swelling, or redness.

What to Do: Discontinue the drug and consult your doctor. If this drug is accidentally ingested, call your doctor, emergency medical services (EMS), or the nearest poison control center immediately.

▼ INTERACTIONS

DRUG INTERACTIONS
Use of this medicine with skin-peeling agents such as salicylic acid, sulfur, tretinoin, or resorcinol can cause excessive skin irritation. Consult your doctor if you take an oral contraceptive, or if you are using any other prescription or nonprescription medication for acne, or if you use medicated cosmetics or abrasive skin cleaners.

FOOD INTERACTIONS
See below.

DISEASE INTERACTIONS
A history of allergy to cinnamon and foods containing benzoic acid increases the chances of developing an allergic skin rash to benzoyl peroxide. Be sure to notify your doctor if you have either of these allergies. Consult your doctor before you use benzoyl peroxide if you have any skin condition other than acne.

BETA-CAROTENE

Available in: Capsules, tablets
Available as Generic? Yes
Drug Class: Dietary supplement

▼ USAGE INFORMATION

WHY IT'S TAKEN
Beta-carotene is a natural source of vitamin A. While most Americans get sufficient amounts of vitamin A in their diet, beta-carotene may be prescribed as a dietary supplement for people with certain medical conditions that increase the need for the vitamin. Such conditions include cystic fibrosis, long-term chronic illness, chronic diarrhea, and intestinal malabsorption. A profound deficiency of vitamin A (which occurs very rarely) can lead to night blindness. It may also lead to skin problems, dry eyes and eye infections, and slowed growth. In larger doses beta-carotene may also be recommended to reduce the severity of photosensitive reactions (heightened sensitivity to sunlight) that occur in patients with a rare inherited disorder known as erythopoietic protoporphyria. Beta-carotene is an antioxidant that has been prescribed to prevent atherosclerosis and coronary heart disease, but beta-carotene supplements did not reduce the incidence of heart attacks in three large clinical trials.

HOW IT WORKS
Approximately half of ingested beta-carotene is converted to vitamin A in the intestine. The rest is absorbed unchanged and is stored in various tissues, especially fat.

▼ DOSAGE GUIDELINES

RANGE AND FREQUENCY
As a dietary supplement— Adults and teenagers: 6 to 15 mg a day. Children: 3 to 6 mg a day. To treat erythopoietic porphyria—30 to 300 mg a day.

ONSET OF EFFECT
Unknown.

DURATION OF ACTION
Unknown.

DIETARY ADVICE
It is best taken with meals.

STORAGE
Store in a tightly sealed container kept away from heat, moisture, and direct light. Do not refrigerate beta-carotene, and keep it from freezing.

MISSED DOSE
There is no danger in doubling the next dose if you miss a scheduled dose.

STOPPING THE DRUG
Take it as recommended. If you are using beta-carotene for a specific medical condition, the decision to stop taking it should be made in consultation with your doctor.

PROLONGED USE
No known problems.

▼ PRECAUTIONS

Over 60: No special precautions are warranted.

Driving and Hazardous Work: No precautions are necessary.

Alcohol: No special precautions are necessary.

Pregnancy: Beta-carotene has not been studied in pregnant women, but no problems with fertility or pregnancy have been reported in women taking up to 30 mg of beta-carotene a day. The effects of higher daily doses are unknown.

Breast Feeding: Beta-carotene may pass into breast milk, although problems have not been documented with the intake of normal recommended amounts. Consult your doctor for advice.

Infants and Children: No problems have been reported with the intake of beta-carotene in recommended amounts.

Special Concerns: Beta-carotene is found in carrots, dark-green leafy vegetables such as spinach and lettuce, tomatoes, sweet potatoes, broccoli, cantaloupe, and winter squash. Be sure to eat a proper, balanced diet to obtain adequate amounts of beta-carotene from foods. Some fat is needed so that the body can absorb beta-carotene. Beta-carotene is safer than vitamin A, which, in high doses, can damage the liver. If high levels of vitamin A are present, less beta-carotene is converted to vitamin A by the body.

OVERDOSE
Symptoms: None have been reported.

What to Do: An overdose of beta-carotene is unlikely to be dangerous. Emergency instructions do not apply.

▼ INTERACTIONS

DRUG INTERACTIONS
Consult your doctor for specific advice if you are taking cholestyramine or colestipol (cholesterol-lowering drugs), mineral oil, neomycin (an antibiotic), or vitamin E.

FOOD INTERACTIONS
No known food interactions.

DISEASE INTERACTIONS
If you have any medical problems, consult your doctor before taking beta-carotene. Large doses of beta-carotene may cause complications in patients with liver disease or kidney disease.

≡ SIDE EFFECTS ≡

SERIOUS
No serious side effects are associated with beta-carotene.

COMMON
Yellowing of the palms, hands, or soles of feet, and, in some cases, the face.

LESS COMMON
No less common side effects are associated with the use of beta-carotene.

BIOTIN

Available in: Capsules, tablets
Available as Generic? Yes
Drug Class: Vitamin

▼ USAGE INFORMATION

WHY IT'S TAKEN

Biotin is a vitamin found naturally in various foods (see Dietary Advice for more information). While most people get sufficient amounts of it in their diet, biotin may be needed as a dietary supplement for people on inadequate or unusual diets or with medical conditions that increase the need for it. Such conditions include a genetic deficiency of the enzyme (biotinidase) needed by the body to utilize biotin, intestinal malabsorption, seborrheic dermatitis in infancy, and an inability to absorb biotin as a result of surgical removal of the stomach. Biotin deficiency may lead to dermatitis, hair loss, high blood cholesterol levels, and heart problems.

HOW IT WORKS

Biotin is one of the B vitamins necessary for the formation of glucose and fatty acids, and for the metabolism of amino acids and carbohydrates. B vitamins are particularly crucial to the proper functioning of the cardiovascular and nervous systems.

▼ DOSAGE GUIDELINES

RANGE AND FREQUENCY

No recommended daily allowances (RDAs) have been established for biotin. The following daily intakes are advised. Adults and teenagers: 30 to 100 micrograms (mcg). Children ages 7 to 10 years: 30 mcg. Children ages 4 to 6 years: 25 mcg daily. Birth to 3 years: 10 to 20 mcg.

ONSET OF EFFECT

Unknown.

DURATION OF ACTION

Unknown.

DIETARY ADVICE

Biotin can be taken with or between meals. Foods that contain biotin include cauliflower, liver, salmon, carrots, bananas, cereals, yeast, and soy flour. Biotin content is reduced when food is cooked or preserved.

STORAGE

Store in a tightly sealed container protected from heat, moisture, and direct light.

MISSED DOSE

Take it as soon as you remember.

≡ SIDE EFFECTS ≡

SERIOUS

No serious side effects are associated with recommended doses of biotin. However, check with your doctor if you notice anything unusual while you are taking it.

COMMON

No common side effects are associated with recommended doses.

LESS COMMON

No less-common side effects have been reported.

STOPPING THE DRUG

If you are taking biotin for a vitamin deficiency or medical problem, take it as prescribed for the full treatment period.

PROLONGED USE

When biotin is prescribed to overcome a deficiency, periodic monitoring of biotin levels in the blood may be required.

▼ PRECAUTIONS

Over 60: No problems are expected in older persons taking recommended doses of biotin.

Driving and Hazardous Work: The use of biotin should not impair your ability to perform such tasks safely.

Alcohol: No special precautions are necessary.

Pregnancy: No problems are expected with the intake of recommended doses of biotin during pregnancy.

Breast Feeding: No problems are expected with the intake of recommended doses of biotin during breast feeding.

Infants and Children: No problems are expected with recommended doses.

Special Concerns: Some drastic weight-reducing diets may may not supply enough biotin. Consult your doctor for specific advice. Biotin is generally available as part of a multivitamin complex.

OVERDOSE

Symptoms: No cases of overdose have been reported.

What to Do: Emergency instructions not applicable.

▼ INTERACTIONS

DRUG INTERACTIONS

There are no known drug interactions associated with biotin.

FOOD INTERACTIONS

No known food interactions.

DISEASE INTERACTIONS

None reported.

BISACODYL

Available in: Tablets, powder, suppositories
Available as Generic? Yes
Drug Class: Stimulant laxative

▼ USAGE INFORMATION

WHY IT'S TAKEN
To relieve short-term consti-pation or to clear the bowel before rectal or bowel exami-nation, surgery, or childbirth.

HOW IT WORKS
Bisacodyl increases the vol-ume of fluid in the intestines to stimulate passage of the stool. It also acts on the smooth muscle of the intes-tine to increase contractions.

▼ DOSAGE GUIDELINES

RANGE AND FREQUENCY
For constipation—Adults and teenagers: Tablets: 10 to 15 mg at bedtime. Children age 6 and older: 5 mg before breakfast. Swallow tablets whole; do not chew. For medical examination—Adults and teenagers: Up to 30 mg orally, or 10 mg given rectally before examination. Children age 6 and older: 5 mg orally or rectally, before breakfast.

ONSET OF EFFECT
Tablets: Within 6 to 12 hours. Suppositories: Within 15 to 60 minutes.

DURATION OF ACTION
Variable.

DIETARY ADVICE
Take the tablet on an empty stomach for rapid effect. Increase intake of fluids and dietary fiber.

STORAGE
Store in a tightly sealed con-tainer and keep away from heat, moisture, and direct light.

MISSED DOSE
Take the missed dose as soon as you remember, unless it is almost time for your next dose. In that case, skip the missed dose and resume your regular dosage schedule. Do not double the next dose.

STOPPING THE DRUG
Take it as prescribed for the full treatment period. How-ever, you may stop taking the drug if you are feeling better before the scheduled end of the therapy.

PROLONGED USE
Do not use this medicine for more than one week unless your doctor prescribes it.

▼ PRECAUTIONS

Over 60: Excessive use of this drug by an older person can cause loss of body fluid leading to weakness and lack of coordination.

Driving and Hazardous Work: Do not drive or engage in hazardous work until you determine how the medicine affects you.

Alcohol: Avoid alcohol while taking this drug.

Pregnancy: Bisacodyl is not usually used during preg-nancy, except immediately before delivery. Consult your doctor for advice.

Breast Feeding: Bisacodyl may pass into breast milk. Consult your doctor for spe-cific advice.

Infants and Children: Do not give this medicine to a child under 6 without your doctor's approval. Do not give this medicine to a child who refuses to have a bowel movement. It may result in a painful bowel movement, which will make the child resist even more.

Special Concerns: Remember that chronic use of bisacodyl or any laxative can lead to laxative dependence. You should consume adequate amounts of fiber in your diet, sources of which include bran or whole-grain cereals, fruit, and vegetables.

OVERDOSE
Symptoms: Weakness, increased sweating, lower abdominal pain, muscle cramps, irregular heartbeat.

What to Do: An overdose of bisacodyl is unlikely to be life-threatening. However, if someone takes a much larger dose than prescribed, seek medical assistance right away.

▼ INTERACTIONS

DRUG INTERACTIONS
Be sure to tell your doctor about any other drugs you are taking, especially antacids. Do not take an antacid within 2 hours of taking this drug.

FOOD INTERACTIONS
Do not drink milk within 2 hours of taking this drug.

DISEASE INTERACTIONS
Caution is advised when tak-ing bisacodyl. Consult your doctor if you have very severe constipation, severe pain in the stomach or lower abdomen, cramping, bloating, nausea, or unexplained rectal bleeding. Failure to produce a bowel movement or the pres-ence of rectal bleeding may indicate a serious medical condition.

⬇ SIDE EFFECTS ⬇

SERIOUS
Severe stomach pain, laxative dependence. Call your doc-tor immediately.

COMMON
Abdominal cramping, burning sensation in the rectum (with suppository), diarrhea.

LESS COMMON
Nausea; vomiting; muscle weakness; rectal pain, bleeding, burning, or itching. If you have a sudden change in bowel habits that lasts longer than 2 weeks, consult your doctor.

BISMUTH SUBSALICYLATE

Available in: Tablets, oral suspension
Available as Generic? Yes
Drug Class: Antidiarrheal/antacid

▼ USAGE INFORMATION

WHY IT'S TAKEN
To treat heartburn, acid indigestion, diarrhea, and duodenal ulcers, and to help prevent traveler's diarrhea.

HOW IT WORKS
Bismuth subsalicylate stimulates the passage of fluid and electrolytes across the wall of the intestinal tract, and binds or neutralizes the toxins of some bacteria, rendering them nontoxic. It decreases intestinal inflammation and increases the activity of intestinal muscles and lining.

▼ DOSAGE GUIDELINES

RANGE AND FREQUENCY
Adults –For acid indigestion or mild diarrhea: 2 tablets or 2 tablespoons of liquid every 30 to 60 minutes, to a maximum of 16 doses daily of the regular-strength drug for no more than 2 days. Children ages 9 to 12–1 tablet or 1 tablespoon every 30 to 60 minutes, to a maximum of 8 doses daily of the regular-strength drug for no more than 2 days. Children ages 6 to 9–2 teaspoons every 30 to 60 minutes, to a maximum of 16 doses daily of the regular-strength drug for no more than 2 days. Children under age 3–Consult your pediatrician. Tablets are not recommended for children under the age of 9.

ONSET OF EFFECT
Within 30 to 60 minutes.

DURATION OF ACTION
Unknown.

DIETARY ADVICE
A mild diet is recommended when you're recovering from diarrhea. Bananas, rice, applesauce, and plain toast are good choices. Be sure to get plenty of fluids.

STORAGE
Store in a tightly sealed container away from heat and direct light. Keep liquid forms of bismuth subsalicylate refrigerated, but do not allow the medicine to freeze.

MISSED DOSE
Take it as soon as you remember. If it is near the time for the next dose, skip the missed dose and resume your regular dosage schedule. Do not double the next dose.

STOPPING THE DRUG
Take it as recommended for the full treatment period. However, you may stop taking the drug if you feel better before the scheduled end of therapy.

PROLONGED USE
Prolonged use of this medicine may cause constipation. Consult your physician if relief is not achieved within two days.

▼ PRECAUTIONS

Over 60: Adverse reactions may be more likely and more severe in older patients.

Driving and Hazardous Work: Do not drive or engage in hazardous work until you determine how this medicine affects you.

Alcohol: Alcohol intake should be limited.

Pregnancy: Regular use of this medicine late in pregnancy may harm the fetus or cause delivery problems. Consult your doctor about taking it if you are pregnant or plan to become pregnant.

Breast Feeding: Bismuth subsalicylate passes into breast milk; avoid or discontinue use while nursing.

Infants and Children: Consult your doctor before giving this medicine to a child or teenager who has or is recovering from chicken pox or flu.

Special Concerns: Do not take bismuth subsalicylate if you are allergic to aspirin or another salicylate, or if you are taking an anticoagulant, or a medicine for diabetes or gout. Do not swallow tablets whole. Crush, chew, or allow the tablets to dissolve in the mouth.

OVERDOSE
Symptoms: Seizures, confusion, rapid or deep breathing, hearing loss or ringing or buzzing in the ears, severe excitability or nervousness, severe drowsiness, loss of consciousness.

What to Do: Call your doctor, emergency medical services (EMS), or the nearest poison control center immediately.

▼ INTERACTIONS

DRUG INTERACTIONS
Consult your doctor for specific advice if you are taking anticoagulants, aspirin and other salicylates, oral diabetes medicine, heparin, probenecid, thrombolytic agents, oral tetracycline, or sulfinpyrazone.

FOOD INTERACTIONS
No known food interactions.

DISEASE INTERACTIONS
Caution is advised when using bismuth subsalicylate. Before taking this drug, tell your doctor if you have a history of allergies, diabetes, kidney disease, dehydration, stomach ulcers, dysentery, gout, or a bleeding problem.

≡ SIDE EFFECTS ≡

SERIOUS
Ringing in the ears. Call your doctor immediately.

COMMON
Black stools, darkening of the tongue.

LESS COMMON
Nausea, vomiting (with high doses), abdominal pain, increased sweating, muscle weakness, hearing loss, thirst, confusion, dizziness, vision problems, trouble breathing. Discontinue the medicine and call your physician right away.

BROMPHENIRAMINE MALEATE

Available in: Capsules, tablets, extended-release tablets, elixir
Available as Generic? Yes
Drug Class: Antihistamine

▼ USAGE INFORMATION

WHY IT'S TAKEN
To prevent or relieve symptoms of hay fever, allergies, itching skin, or hives.

HOW IT WORKS
The drug brompheniramine blocks the effects of histamine, a chemical substance released by the body that causes swelling, itching, sneezing, watery eyes, hives, and other symptoms of an allergic reaction.

▼ DOSAGE GUIDELINES

RANGE AND FREQUENCY
Capsules, tablets, elixir—Adults and teenagers: 4 mg every 4 to 6 hours. Children ages 6 to 12: 2 mg every 4 to 6 hours. Children ages 2 to 6: 1 mg every 4 to 6 hours. Extended-release tablets—Adults: 8 mg every 8 to 12 hours, or 12 mg every 12 hours. Children age 6 and older: 8 or 12 mg every 12 hours.

ONSET OF EFFECT
15 to 60 minutes.

DURATION OF ACTION
3 to 6 hours when taken in regular form; 8 to 12 hours for extended-release tablets.

DIETARY ADVICE
Take it with food or milk to minimize stomach upset.

STORAGE
Store in a sealed container away from heat and light.

MISSED DOSE
Take it as soon as you remember. If it is near the time for the next dose, skip the missed dose and resume your regular dosage schedule. Do not double the next dose.

STOPPING THE DRUG
Take as recommended for the full treatment period, but you may stop if you feel better before the scheduled end of therapy, or take as needed.

PROLONGED USE
No special concerns.

▼ PRECAUTIONS

Over 60: Older persons are more sensitive to anti-histamine side effects, particularly confusion, dizziness, drowsiness, restlessness, irritability, nightmares, and dry mouth, nose, and throat.

Driving and Hazardous Work: Brompheniramine can make you feel tired and lessen your concentration. Do not drive or engage in hazardous work until you determine how the drug affects you.

Alcohol: Alcohol increases the likelihood and the severity of side effects like drowsiness and confusion.

Pregnancy: Animals studies suggest that brompheniramine has no adverse effect on fetal development, but human studies have not been done. Before taking this drug, consult your doctor if you are pregnant or are planning to become pregnant.

Breast Feeding: Brompheniramine passes into breast milk; avoid or discontinue use while breast feeding.

Infants and Children: Brompheniramine should be given to children age 6 and under only upon a doctor's recommendation.

Special Concerns: Do not break, crush, or chew the capsules or the extended-release tablets.

OVERDOSE
Symptoms: Seizures, loss of consciousness, hallucinations, severe drowsiness.

What to Do: The patient should be made to vomit immediately, using ipecac syrup. If he or she is unconscious, the patient should be taken to a hospital emergency room immediately.

▼ INTERACTIONS

DRUG INTERACTIONS
MAO inhibitors can increase the sedative effects of brompheniramine. Central nervous system depressants such as alcohol, sedatives, or narcotics should be taken only if approved by a doctor.

FOOD INTERACTIONS
No known food interactions.

DISEASE INTERACTIONS
Before taking brompheniramine, consult your doctor if you wear contact lenses or you have glaucoma, prostate enlargement, difficulty with urination, or dryness of the mouth or eyes.

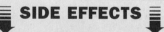

SIDE EFFECTS

SERIOUS
Bleeding problems; small, red pinpoints on the skin; fever; extreme fatigue; bleeding ulcers in the rectum, mouth, and vagina; reduced white blood cell count (rare).

COMMON
Drowsiness; unusual excitability; dry mouth, nose, or throat. Symptoms of drowsiness tend to subside after a few days' use as your body adjusts to the drug.

LESS COMMON
Vision changes, loss of appetite, dizziness, painful or difficult urination, less tolerance for contact lenses.

BUTOCONAZOLE NITRATE

Femstat 3

Available in: Vaginal cream
Available as Generic? No
Drug Class: Antifungal

▼ USAGE INFORMATION

WHY IT'S TAKEN
To treat fungal (yeast) infections of the vagina.

HOW IT WORKS
Butoconazole prevents fungal organisms from producing vital substances required for growth and function. This drug is effective only for infections caused by fungal organisms. It will not work for bacterial or viral infections.

▼ DOSAGE GUIDELINES

RANGE AND FREQUENCY
Nonpregnant women and teenagers: 5 g (1 applicatorful) of cream inserted with an applicator into the vagina at bedtime for 3 consecutive days. Pregnant women and teenagers: After third month, 5 g (1 applicatorful) of cream inserted with an applicator into the vagina at bedtime for 6 consecutive days.

ONSET OF EFFECT
Unknown.

DURATION OF ACTION
Unknown.

DIETARY ADVICE
Butoconazole can be applied without regard to diet.

STORAGE
Store in a tightly sealed container away from moisture, heat, and direct light. Do not allow it to freeze.

MISSED DOSE
Insert it as soon as you remember. If it is near the time for the next dose, skip the missed dose and resume your regular dosage schedule.

STOPPING THE DRUG
Use the medicine as directed for the full treatment period, even if you begin to feel better before the scheduled end of therapy. Recurrence of the infection is likely if you stop before the full treatment period is complete.

PROLONGED USE
Butoconazole is generally prescribed for short-term therapy (3 to 6 days).

▼ PRECAUTIONS

Over 60: No special problems are expected.

Driving and Hazardous Work: The use of butoconazole should not adversely affect your ability to perform such tasks safely.

Alcohol: No special precautions are necessary.

Pregnancy: Studies on the use of butoconazole during the first 3 months (trimester) of pregnancy have not been done. No adverse effects while using it during the second or third trimesters have been reported.

Breast Feeding: No problems are expected. Consult your doctor about using this medicine while nursing.

Infants and Children: Studies on the use of butoconazole in children have not been done. Consult your pediatrician for specific advice.

Special Concerns: The drug may be used with oral contraceptives and antibiotic therapy. Sanitary napkins should be used to prevent staining of clothing. The affected area should be kept cool and dry. The patient should wear loose-fitting cotton clothing and freshly laundered cotton underwear or pantyhose with a cotton crotch. Avoid underwear made from materials that block air. Do not sit for a long time in a wet bathing suit. Avoid feminine hygiene sprays. Wash area daily with unscented soap and dry thoroughly with a clean towel. Tampons should not be used during therapy. The patient's sexual partner should wear a condom during intercourse and should consult a doctor if penile redness, itching, or discomfort occurs. Do not stop using this medicine during your menstrual period. After urination or a bowel movement, cleanse by wiping the area from front to back to prevent reinfection.

OVERDOSE
Symptoms: An overdose with butoconazole is unlikely.

What to Do: If someone should swallow a large amount of butoconazole, call your doctor, emergency medical services (EMS), or the nearest poison control center immediately.

▼ INTERACTIONS

DRUG INTERACTIONS
Tell your doctor if you are using any other prescription or OTC vaginal medication.

FOOD INTERACTIONS
No food interactions have been reported.

DISEASE INTERACTIONS
No disease interactions have been reported.

≡ SIDE EFFECTS ≡

▼ SERIOUS ▼
Vaginal itching, burning, discharge, or irritation not present prior to treatment. Call your doctor as soon as possible.

COMMON
No common side effects are associated with the use of butoconazole.

LESS COMMON
Headache, stomach cramps or pain, irritation or burning of sexual partner's penis.

CAFFEINE

Available in: Tablets, extended-release capsules
Available as Generic? Yes
Drug Class: Central nervous system stimulant

▼ USAGE INFORMATION

WHY IT'S TAKEN
To restore mental alertness.

HOW IT WORKS
Caffeine acts as a stimulant to all levels of the central nervous system.

▼ DOSAGE GUIDELINES

RANGE AND FREQUENCY
Tablets: 100 to 200 mg; repeat after 3 or 4 hours if needed. Extended-release capsules: 200 to 250 mg; can be repeated after 3 or 4 hours if needed. Citrated caffeine: 65 to 325 mg, 3 times a day as needed. Take no more than 1,000 mg a day.

ONSET OF EFFECT
Unknown.

DURATION OF ACTION
Unknown.

DIETARY ADVICE
Take it with food to minimize stomach upset.

STORAGE
Store in a tightly sealed container away from heat and direct light. Keep away from moisture and extremes in temperature.

MISSED DOSE
Take it as soon as you remember. If it is near the time for the next dose, skip the missed dose and resume your regular dosage schedule. Do not double the next dose.

STOPPING THE DRUG
The decision to stop taking the drug should be made by your doctor.

PROLONGED USE
Caffeine is not intended for prolonged use.

▼ PRECAUTIONS

Over 60: No special problems are expected.

Driving and Hazardous Work: The use of caffeine should not impair your ability to perform such tasks safely.

Alcohol: No special precautions are necessary.

Pregnancy: Large doses can cause miscarriage, delay the growth of the fetus, or cause problems with the heart rhythm of the fetus. No more than 300 mg of caffeine (the amount in 3 cups of coffee) should be consumed daily during pregnancy.

Breast Feeding: Caffeine passes into breast milk; caution is advised. Consult your doctor for specific advice.

Infants and Children: Caffeine is not recommended for use by children under the age of 12.

Special Concerns: To prevent insomnia, do not take caffeine or drink caffeine-containing beverages too close to bedtime. After you stop taking caffeine, especially if you stop abruptly, you may experience anxiety, dizziness, headache, irritability, muscle tension, nausea, nervousness, stuffy nose, and unusual fatigue. Consult your doctor if you suffer from any of these symptoms.

OVERDOSE
Symptoms: Stomach or abdominal pains, agitation, anxiety, excitement, restlessness, confusion, delirium, seizures. A very large overdose can cause an irregular heartbeat; seeing zig-zag flashes of light; frequent urination; increased sensitivity to touch; muscle twitching; nausea and vomiting, sometimes with blood; insomnia; and ringing in the ears.

What to Do: An overdose of caffeine is unlikely to be life-threatening. However, if someone takes a much larger dose than directed, call your doctor, emergency medical services (EMS), or the nearest poison control right away.

▼ INTERACTIONS

DRUG INTERACTIONS
Call your doctor for specific advice if you are also taking central nervous system stimulants; MAO inhibitors; amantadine; ciprofloxacin and norfloxacin (antibiotics); cold, sinus, hay fever, or allergy medications; asthma medicine; pemoline; amphetamines; nabilone; methylphenidate; or chlophedianol.

FOOD INTERACTIONS
Do not drink large amounts of caffeine-containing beverages like coffee, tea, soft drinks, cocoa, or chocolate milk.

DISEASE INTERACTIONS
Caution is advised when taking caffeine. Consult your doctor if you have any of the following: anxiety, panic attacks, heart disease, high blood pressure, agoraphobia (fear of open places), or insomnia. Use of caffeine may cause complications in patients with liver disease, since this organ works to remove the medication from the body.

≡ SIDE EFFECTS ≡

⬇ SERIOUS ⬇
Diarrhea, insomnia, dizziness, rapid heartbeat, severe nausea, vomiting, irritability, unusual agitation, tremors. Call your doctor immediately.

COMMON
Mild nausea or jitters.

LESS COMMON
There are no less-common side effects associated with the use of caffeine.

CALAMINE

BRAND NAME

Calamox

Available in: Lotion, ointment
Available as Generic? Yes
Drug Class: Topical anti-itching agent; astringent

▼ USAGE INFORMATION

WHY IT'S TAKEN
To relieve the itching, pain, and discomfort of skin irritations, such as those caused by poison ivy, poison oak, and poison sumac. Calamine will also dry the oozing and weeping of skin eruptions caused by poison ivy, poison oak, and poison sumac.

HOW IT WORKS
The exact mechanism of action is unknown; calamine appears to have natural soothing properties.

▼ DOSAGE GUIDELINES

RANGE AND FREQUENCY
Apply calamine to the affected area of skin as often as needed. To use the lotion, shake it well to start. Then moisten a wad of cotton with the lotion and use the cotton to apply the lotion to the affected area of skin. Allow the lotion to dry on the skin. To use the ointment, gently rub just enough ointment into the skin to lightly cover the affected area.

ONSET OF EFFECT
Within 1 hour.

DURATION OF ACTION
Unknown.

DIETARY ADVICE
Calamine can be used without regard to diet.

STORAGE
Store in a tightly sealed container away from heat and direct light. Do not refrigerate calamine or allow the medication to freeze.

MISSED DOSE
If you are using calamine on a fixed schedule, apply the missed dose as soon as you remember. If it is close to the next dose, skip the missed dose and resume your regular dosage schedule. Do not use more lotion or ointment than necessary per application.

STOPPING THE DRUG
Apply calamine as recommended for as long as your symptoms last.

PROLONGED USE
Call your doctor if you have a skin condition that does not improve or gets worse after 7 days of treatment with calamine.

▼ PRECAUTIONS

Over 60: No special problems have been documented in older patients.

Driving and Hazardous Work: Use of calamine should not impair your ability to perform such tasks safely.

Alcohol: No special precautions are necessary.

Pregnancy: No problems during pregnancy have been documented.

Breast Feeding: Calamine may be used safely while nursing; no problems that affect the baby during breast feeding have been documented.

Infants and Children: Studies on the use of calamine on infants and children have not been done; however, no pediatric-specific problems have been documented.

Special Concerns: Calamine is for external use only. Do not swallow it. Do not use calamine on the eyes or mucous membranes, such as the inside of the mouth, nose, genitals, or anal area. Ingestion of calamine has been reported to cause gastritis (inflammation of the stomach lining) and vomiting. Milk or antacids may be used to treat these symptoms.

OVERDOSE
Symptoms: None.

What to Do: No emergency instructions are applicable, since no cases of overdose have been reported. However, if someone accidentally ingests calamine, seek medical assistance right away.

▼ INTERACTIONS

DRUG INTERACTIONS
No drug interactions with calamine have been reported. However, you should tell your doctor if you are using any other prescription or over-the-counter medication to treat the same area of skin as calamine.

FOOD INTERACTIONS
No known food interactions.

DISEASE INTERACTIONS
No disease interactions with calamine have been documented. However, tell your doctor if you have any other skin condition.

≣ SIDE EFFECTS ≣

SERIOUS
No serious side effects are associated with calamine.

COMMON
No common side effects are associated with calamine.

LESS COMMON
Rash, irritation, or sensitivity of the treated area that was not present prior to beginning therapy. Call your doctor promptly if such symptoms persist.

CALCIUM

Available in: Capsules, oral suspension, tablets, chewable tablets, liquid
Available as Generic? Yes
Drug Class: Antihypocalcemic; dietary supplement; antacid

▼ USAGE INFORMATION

WHY IT'S TAKEN
To ensure adequate calcium intake in those who do not get sufficient amounts by diet alone. Calcium is essential to many body functions, including the transmission of nerve impulses, the regulation of muscle contraction and relaxation (including of the heart), blood clotting, and various metabolic activities. Calcium is necessary for maintaining strong bones as well and is commonly recommended to prevent and treat postmenopausal osteoporosis (bone thinning). Vitamin D supplements, which aid in the absorption of calcium from the intestine, are often used along with calcium supplements to prevent or treat osteoporosis. (Indeed, some calcium supplement tablets contain vitamin D.) Calcium is also prescribed for individuals with persistently low levels of calcium in the blood (hypocalcemia) caused, for example, by low blood levels of parathyroid hormone (hypoparathyroidism).

HOW IT WORKS
Calcium supplements compensate for inadequate dietary intake of this essential mineral. Supplementary calcium is available in the form of calcium carbonate (the most common and inexpensive), calcium citrate (the best absorbed, but relatively expensive), calcium phosphate, calcium lactate, or calcium gluconate. Because calcium carbonate and phosphate supplements are hard to absorb, other calcium products are preferable for individuals with low gastric (stomach) acid secretion.

▼ DOSAGE GUIDELINES

RANGE AND FREQUENCY
Optimal daily calcium intakes–Ages 0 to 6 months: 210 mg. Ages 6 months to 1 year: 270 mg. Ages 1 to 3 years: 500 mg. Ages 4 to 8 years: 800 mg. Ages 9 to 18 years: 1,300 mg. Ages 19 to 50 years: 1,000 mg. Age 51 and older: 1,200. For pregnant or breast-feeding women, under 19 years: 1,300 mg; ages 19 to 50 years: 1,000 mg. When you figure your calcium intake, be sure to include dietary calcium as well as the supplements. Calcium itself constitutes only a fraction of any calcium-containing pill. For example, calcium accounts for only 40% of the weight of a calcium carbonate tablet. Thus, a 500 mg tablet of calcium carbonate provides only 200 mg of calcium.

ONSET OF EFFECT
Unknown.

DURATION OF ACTION
For as long as the supplement is taken.

DIETARY ADVICE
Calcium carbonate and calcium phosphate supplements are best absorbed if taken 60 to 90 minutes after meals. Take with 1 full glass (8 oz) of water or juice. Follow all special dietary guidelines your doctor recommends.

STORAGE
Store in a tightly sealed container protected from heat, moisture, and direct light.

MISSED DOSE
If you are taking a calcium supplement on a regular basis and miss a dose, take it as soon as you remember, then resume your regular dosage schedule.

STOPPING THE DRUG
The decision to stop taking calcium supplements should be made in consultation with your doctor.

PROLONGED USE
Adverse effects are more likely to occur if supplements are taken in doses greater than 2,000 to 2,500 mg a day for a long period of time. Your doctor should regularly check your blood calcium levels if you are taking calcium supplements to treat low blood calcium (hypocalcemia).

▼ PRECAUTIONS

Over 60: No special problems are expected.

Driving and Hazardous Work: Calcium supplements should have no effect on your ability to perform such tasks safely.

Alcohol: To ensure proper absorption of calcium, consume alcohol in moderation only (2 drinks per day).

Pregnancy: It is crucial to take in enough calcium during pregnancy and to maintain those levels throughout pregnancy, preferably through diet alone. However, excessive calcium intake during pregnancy may be harmful to the mother or fetus and should be avoided.

≡ SIDE EFFECTS ≡

SERIOUS
Serious side effects are associated with excessively high doses (see Overdose).

COMMON
No common side effects are associated with recommended doses of calcium.

LESS COMMON
Constipation, diarrhea, drowsiness, loss of appetite, dry mouth, and muscle weakness are some of the symptoms that could result if blood levels of calcium are too high (hypercalcemia).

Breast Feeding: Excessive amounts of this supplement taken while nursing may be harmful to the mother or infant and should be avoided.

Infants and Children: No special problems expected.

OVERDOSE

Symptoms: Early symptoms: Constipation (especially in children), diarrhea, dry mouth, increased thirst and increased frequency of urination, loss of appetite, persistent headache, metallic taste, nausea and vomiting, unusual fatigue.

Advanced symptoms: Bone and muscle pain, irregular heartbeat, persistent itching, extreme drowsiness, mental changes. Severe calcium toxicity may be fatal.

What to Do: Call your doctor, emergency medical services (EMS), or the nearest poison control center immediately.

▼ INTERACTIONS

DRUG INTERACTIONS
Consult your doctor for specific advice if you are taking other calcium-containing preparations, cellulose sodium phosphate, digitalis drugs, etidronate, gallium nitrate, phenytoin, or tetracycline antibiotics. Combined use of calcium supplements with thiazide diuretics or vitamin D may lead to excessively high calcium levels.

FOOD INTERACTIONS
Excessive protein consumption can increase the excretion of calcium in the urine. In meals preceding calcium consumption, avoid spinach and rhubarb (high in oxalic acid), and bran and whole cereals (high in phytic acid), since these substances may interfere with calcium absorption.

DISEASE INTERACTIONS
Consult your doctor if you have frequent episodes of diarrhea, any stomach or intestinal problems, heart disease, sarcoidosis, kidney disease, or kidney stones.

CAPSAICIN

BRAND NAMES

Axsain, Zostrix

Available in: Cream
Available as Generic? Yes
Drug Class: Analgesic

▼ USAGE INFORMATION

WHY IT'S TAKEN
To relieve neuralgia—pain in the nerve endings near the surface of the skin. Capsaicin is commonly recommended for neuralgia associated with shingles, an acutely painful condition caused by infection with the varicella zoster virus, the same organism that causes chicken pox. Capsaicin is also a treatment for mild to moderate arthritis, diabetic neuropathy (pain caused by nerve cell damage that occurs as a complication of diabetes), and postoperative pain.

HOW IT WORKS
When applied topically, capsaicin (a derivative of hot peppers) appears to reduce the amount of a natural chemical known as substance P, which is present in painful joints. Substance P is believed to be involved in two processes central to arthritis: the release of enzymes that produce inflammation and the transmission of pain impulses from the joints to the central nervous system. By blocking the production and release of substance P, capsaicin can reduce the pain associated with arthritis as well as dampen the transmission of pain messages to the brain.

▼ DOSAGE GUIDELINES

RANGE AND FREQUENCY
Apply a small amount to the affected area up to 4 times a day. Do not apply to broken or irritated skin. If the use of a bandage is recommended, do not apply it too tightly.

ONSET OF EFFECT
Therapeutic pain response is usually achieved in 1 to 2 weeks but may take as long as 4 weeks.

DURATION OF ACTION
Up to 6 hours.

DIETARY ADVICE
This medication can be used without regard to diet.

STORAGE
Store in a tightly sealed container away from heat and direct light.

MISSED DOSE
Apply it as soon as you remember. If it is near the time for the next dose, skip the missed dose and resume your regular dosage schedule. Do not double the next dose.

STOPPING THE DRUG
Pain relief will last only as long as capsaicin is used regularly. If you discontinue using the medication and the pain returns, it is safe to resume treatment.

PROLONGED USE
No special problems are expected. Burning and stinging sensations upon application frequently subside with prolonged use. If your condition worsens or does not improve after 1 month, discontinue using capsaicin and consult your doctor.

▼ PRECAUTIONS

Over 60: No special problems are expected.

Driving and Hazardous Work: No problems are expected.

Alcohol: No special precautions are necessary.

Pregnancy: No problems have been reported.

Breast Feeding: No problems are expected.

Infants and Children: Not recommended for use on children under the age of 2. No problems are expected in older children.

Special Concerns: You may not be able to use capsaicin if you are allergic to it or if you have ever had an allergic reaction to hot peppers. Wash your hands thoroughly after applying the cream; if you are using it for arthritis of the hands, wait 30 minutes before washing. It can cause a burning sensation if even small amounts get into the eyes or on other sensitive areas of the body. If you wear contact lenses, be especially cautious. If it does get into your eyes, flush them with water. On other sensitive areas of the body, wash the area with warm (but not hot) soapy water. After applying capsaicin cream, avoid contact with children and pets until you have thoroughly washed your hands.

OVERDOSE
Symptoms: No cases of overdose have been reported.

What to Do: An overdose is unlikely to be life-threatening. However, if someone applies a much larger dose than prescribed, suffers adverse side effects, or accidentally ingests it, call your doctor or the nearest poison control center for advice.

▼ INTERACTIONS

DRUG INTERACTIONS
Capsaicin may alter the action of some drugs or trigger unwanted side effects. Consult your doctor about any other drugs that you take, including over-the-counter medications.

FOOD INTERACTIONS
None are known.

DISEASE INTERACTIONS
Consult your doctor if you have broken or irritated skin, or conditions that may result in broken skin, on the area to be treated.

▤ SIDE EFFECTS ▤

SERIOUS
No serious side effects are associated with capsaicin.

COMMON
Stinging or burning sensation when cream is applied. This should subside with regular use, as your body adjusts to the medication.

LESS COMMON
Skin redness; coughing, sneezing, or shortness of breath if dried residues of the drug are inhaled.

CASTOR OIL

Available in: Oral solution
Available as Generic? Yes
Drug Class: Stimulant laxative

▼ USAGE INFORMATION

WHY IT'S TAKEN
For short-term relief of constipation.

HOW IT WORKS
Castor oil stimulates muscle contractions in the wall of the bowel. These contractions promote the passage of stool.

▼ DOSAGE GUIDELINES

RANGE AND FREQUENCY
The dose will be different for different products. A typical dose is 15 to 60 ml for adults and teenagers. Castor oil should be taken early in the day because the laxative effect is unpredictable and might otherwise interfere with a full night's sleep.

ONSET OF EFFECT
Within 2 to 6 hours.

DURATION OF ACTION
Variable.

DIETARY ADVICE
Laxatives may contain a large amount of sodium or sugar. Regular bowel movements are more likely with a diet that contains an adequate amount of liquid (6 to 8 full 8-oz glasses per day), whole-grain products and bran, fruit, and vegetables.

STORAGE
Store in a tightly sealed container kept away from heat, moisture, and direct light. Refrigerate the liquid form, but do not allow it to freeze.

MISSED DOSE
If you are on a prescribed dosage schedule, take a missed dose as soon as you remember, unless the time for your next scheduled dose is within the next 2 hours. If so, do not take the missed dose. Take your next scheduled dose at the proper time, and resume your regular dosage schedule. Do not double the next dose.

STOPPING THE DRUG
Take it as prescribed for the full treatment period. However, you may stop taking the drug if you are feeling better before the scheduled end of the therapy.

PROLONGED USE
Do not use castor oil for more than 3 to 5 days without informing your physician. Prolonged, excessive use of castor oil may be associated with an increased risk of side effects, including laxative dependence.

▼ PRECAUTIONS

Over 60: Adverse reactions may be more likely and more severe in older patients.

Driving and Hazardous Work: Do not drive or engage in hazardous work until you determine how the medicine affects you.

Alcohol: Avoid alcohol when using this medication.

Pregnancy: Castor oil may cause premature contractions and so should be avoided in pregnant women.

Breast Feeding: Castor oil may be used by nursing mothers.

Infants and Children: Do not give laxatives to children under 6 years of age unless prescribed by a physician.

Special Concerns: Occasional missed bowel movements do not constitute constipation; do not use castor oil under such circumstances. Persistent constipation or difficulty in passing stool is serious and requires evaluation.

OVERDOSE
Symptoms: No cases of overdose with castor oil have been reported.

What to Do: An overdose of castor oil is unlikely to be life-threatening. However, if someone takes a much larger dose than prescribed, contact a physician.

▼ INTERACTIONS

DRUG INTERACTIONS
Do not take a prescription medication within 2 hours of taking a laxative (either before or after), since this may diminish the effects of the prescription drug. Consult your doctor for specific advice if you are taking digitalis drugs or a diuretic.

FOOD INTERACTIONS
No known food interactions.

DISEASE INTERACTIONS
Caution is advised when taking castor oil. Do not use any laxative if you have any of the following: stomach or abdominal pain, especially if accompanied by fever, cramping; abdominal swelling or bloating; nausea or vomiting. Consult your doctor if you are constipated and have any of the following problems: abdominal pain and fever, rectal bleeding, ostomy (an artificial surgical opening in the body to allow the release of urine or feces), diabetes mellitus, heart or kidney disease, or high blood pressure.

≡ SIDE EFFECTS ≡

SERIOUS
Confusion, irregular heartbeat, muscle cramps. Call your doctor immediately.

COMMON
Laxative dependence, skin rashes, stomach cramps, belching, diarrhea, nausea.

LESS COMMON
Fatigue or weakness.

CHARCOAL, ACTIVATED

Available in: Oral suspension, powder, tablets, capsules
Available as Generic? Yes
Drug Class: Antidote

▼ USAGE INFORMATION

WHY IT'S TAKEN
Used as an emergency antidote for treatment of poisonings by most drugs and chemicals; also used to relieve diarrhea or excess gas.

HOW IT WORKS
Activated charcoal prevents the absorption of certain kinds of drugs and chemicals by the body.

▼ DOSAGE GUIDELINES

RANGE AND FREQUENCY
For treatment of poisoning—Oral suspension and powder: Adults and teenagers: 25 to 100 grams (g). Children: 1 g per 2.2 lbs (1 kg) of body weight, or 25 to 50 g. Mix powder with water. Take 1 time only. For treatment of diarrhea—Capsules: Adults and children age 3 and older: 520 mg every 30 to 60 minutes, as needed. Do not take more than 4.16 g per day. For treatment of excess gas—Tablets and capsules: Adults and teenagers: 975 mg to 3.9 g, 3 times a day.

ONSET OF EFFECT
Immediate.

DURATION OF ACTION
Not applicable. Activated charcoal is not absorbed by the body.

DIETARY ADVICE
As an antidote: No special restrictions. To treat diarrhea: It is important to replace the fluid lost by your body and to eat a proper diet. During the first 24 hours, drink plenty of caffeine-free clear liquids like water, broth, ginger ale, and decaffeinated tea. During the second 24 hours you may eat bland foods such as applesauce, bread, crackers, and oatmeal. Avoid caffeine, fried or spicy foods, bran, candy, fruits, and vegetables. These may worsen your condition.

STORAGE
Store in a tightly sealed container away from heat, moisture, and direct light. Premixed suspension can be stored for up to 1 year. Do not allow the liquid form of activated charcoal to freeze.

MISSED DOSE
As an antidote: Not applicable. To treat diarrhea or excess gas: Take it as soon as you remember. If it is near the time for the next dose, skip the missed dose and resume your regular dosage schedule. Do not double the next dose.

STOPPING THE DRUG
As an antidote: Not applicable. To treat diarrhea or excess gas: Take as directed for the full treatment period. However, you may stop taking the drug if you are feeling better before the scheduled end of therapy.

PROLONGED USE
As an antidote: Not applicable. To treat diarrhea: If your diarrhea has not improved or if you have developed a fever after 2 days, call your doctor. To treat excess gas: If your condition has not improved after 3 to 4 days, call your doctor.

▼ PRECAUTIONS

Over 60: No special problems are expected.

Driving and Hazardous Work: The use of activated charcoal should not impair your ability to perform such tasks safely.

Alcohol: No special precautions are necessary.

Pregnancy: Activated charcoal has not been reported to cause problems in an unborn child. Consult your doctor for specific advice.

Breast Feeding: No problems have been reported.

Infants and Children: May be used in infants and children only under strict supervision by a doctor.

Special Concerns: Call your doctor, emergency medical services (EMS), or the nearest poison control center before administering activated charcoal. Charcoal will not be effective if you have been poisoned by swallowing alkalies (lye), petroleum products, strong acids, ethyl or methyl alcohol, iron, boric acid, or lithium. Activated charcoal will not prevent these poisons from being absorbed by the body. If inducing vomiting with ipecac syrup, do so 1 to 2 hours before administering activated charcoal.

OVERDOSE
Symptoms: None expected.

What to Do: Emergency procedures not applicable.

▼ INTERACTIONS

DRUG INTERACTIONS
Activated charcoal may decrease the absorption of any medicine taken within 2 hours of administration. Acetylcysteine and ipecac syrup can decrease the effectiveness of activated charcoal.

FOOD INTERACTIONS
Do not eat chocolate syrup, ice cream, or sherbet with activated charcoal. They will decrease the amount of poison the charcoal can absorb.

DISEASE INTERACTIONS
Caution is advised when taking activated charcoal if you also suffer from dysentery or dehydration.

≡ SIDE EFFECTS ≡

SERIOUS
Swelling or pain in stomach. If this symptom persists, call your doctor immediately.

COMMON
Black, tarry stools.

LESS COMMON
Nausea, constipation. Notify your doctor if any common or less-common side effects persist.

CHLORPHENIRAMINE MALEATE ORAL

Available in: Tablets, sustained-release capsules, syrup
Available as Generic? Yes
Drug Class: Antihistamine

BRAND NAMES

Al-R, Aller-Chlor, Allerid-Od-12, Chlo-Amine, Chlor-100, Chlor-Pro, Chlor-Span-12, Chlor-Trimeton, Chloridamine, Chlorphenamine, Chlortab-8, Com-Time, Cophene-B, Cpc-Carpenters, Halortron, Kloromin, Phenetron, Pyridamal 100, Sinunil-R, Teldrin

▼ USAGE INFORMATION

WHY IT'S TAKEN
To relieve the symptoms of hay fever and other allergies, and for itching skin and hives.

HOW IT WORKS
Chlorpheniramine maleate works by blocking the effects of histamine, a naturally occurring substance that causes swelling, itching, sneezing, watery eyes, hives, and other symptoms of allergic reaction.

▼ DOSAGE GUIDELINES

RANGE AND FREQUENCY
Tablets–Adults: 4 mg, 3 to 4 times per day as needed, for a maximum dose of 24 mg a day. Sustained-release capsules–8 mg every 8 hours, or 12 mg every 12 hours, as needed. Syrup–Children ages 6 to 12: 2 mg, 3 to 4 times a day, not exceeding 12 mg a day. Children ages 2 to 6: 1 mg every 6 hours.

ONSET OF EFFECT
15 to 60 minutes.

DURATION OF ACTION
3 to 6 hours for regular form, 8 to 12 hours for sustained-release capsules.

DIETARY ADVICE
Chlorpheniramine maleate may be taken with food or milk to reduce stomach upset. Use sugarless gum, sugarless sour hard candy, or ice chips to ease dry mouth.

STORAGE
Store in a tightly sealed container away from heat and direct light.

MISSED DOSE
Take it as soon as you remember, up to 2 hours late. If it is more than 2 hours late, skip the missed dose and resume your regular dosage schedule. Do not double the next dose.

STOPPING THE DRUG
You should take it as directed for the full treatment period, but you may stop if you are feeling better before the scheduled end of therapy. Chlorpheniramine may be taken as needed.

PROLONGED USE
No special concerns.

▼ PRECAUTIONS

Over 60: Older persons are more sensitive to antihistamine side effects, particularly confusion, dizziness, drowsiness, restlessness, irritability, nightmares, and dry mouth, nose, and throat.

Driving and Hazardous Work: Do not drive or engage in hazardous work until you determine how the medicine affects you. Use of this drug is a disqualification for piloting aircraft.

Alcohol: Alcohol increases the likelihood and the severity of side effects like drowsiness and confusion.

Pregnancy: In animal studies, no birth defects have been reported. Studies of pregnant women have not been undertaken. Before taking this drug, tell your doctor if you are pregnant or are planning to become pregnant.

Breast Feeding: Chlorpheniramine passes into breast milk; avoid or discontinue use while nursing.

Infants and Children: This drug is not recommended for children under the age of 2.

Special Concerns: Do not break, crush, or chew sustained-release capsules.

OVERDOSE
Symptoms: Marked drowsiness, dilated and sluggish pupils, combativeness, excessive excitability, confusion, loss of coordination, weak pulse, seizures, loss of consciousness.

What to Do: Patient should be made to vomit immediately, using ipecac syrup. If the patient is unconscious, he or she should be taken to the nearest hospital emergency room right away.

▼ INTERACTIONS

DRUG INTERACTIONS
Consult your doctor for specific advice if you are taking anticholinergics, bepridil, medications containing alcohol, or MAO inhibitors.

FOOD INTERACTIONS
No known food interactions.

DISEASE INTERACTIONS
Before taking chlorpheniramine, consult your doctor if you wear contact lenses or if you have glaucoma, prostate enlargement, difficulty with urination, or dry mouth or eyes.

≡ SIDE EFFECTS ≡

SERIOUS
Bleeding problems; small red pinpoints on the skin; fever; extreme fatigue; bleeding ulcers in the rectum, mouth, and vagina; reduced count of white blood cells (rare).

COMMON
Drowsiness; unusual excitability; dry mouth, nose, or throat. Symptoms of drowsiness tend to subside after a few days' use as your body adjusts to the drug.

LESS COMMON
Vision changes, loss of appetite, dizziness, painful or difficult urination, less tolerance for contact lenses.

CIMETIDINE

Available in: Tablets, oral solution, oral suspension
Available as Generic? Yes
Drug Class: Histamine (H2) blocker

▼ USAGE INFORMATION

WHY IT'S TAKEN
To treat ulcers of the stomach and duodenum, as well as other conditions, such as esophagitis (chronic inflammation of the esophagus), and gastroesophageal reflux (backwash of stomach acid into the esophagus, resulting in heartburn).

HOW IT WORKS
Cimetidine blocks the action of histamine (a compound produced in the body's cells), which in turn decreases the stomach's secretion of hydrochloric acid. Once stomach acid production is decreased, the body is better able to heal itself.

▼ DOSAGE GUIDELINES

RANGE AND FREQUENCY
For treatment of acute (symptomatic, bothersome) duodenal or gastric ulcers—Adults and teenagers: Various dosage schedules are used, including 300 mg, 4 times a day, with meals and at bedtime; 400 or 600 mg, 2 times a day; or 800 mg taken once daily at bedtime. For prevention of duodenal ulcers—Adults and teenagers: Usual dose is 300 mg, 2 times a day; another common dosage schedule is 400 mg taken once daily at bedtime. For treatment as needed of heartburn and acid indigestion—Adults and teenagers: 200 mg with water when symptoms start; another 200 mg may be taken within the next 24 hours, for a maximum of 400 mg in a 24-hour period. For treatment of heartburn due to gastroesophageal reflux disease—Adults: 800 to 1,600 mg a day, in 2 to 4 divided doses, for approximately 12 weeks.

ONSET OF EFFECT
Within 1 hour.

DURATION OF ACTION
At least 4 to 5 hours.

DIETARY ADVICE
Avoid foods that cause stomach irritation.

STORAGE
Store away from heat and direct light. Keep the liquid form from freezing.

MISSED DOSE
Take it as soon as you remember. If it is near the time for the next dose, skip the missed dose and resume your regular dosage schedule. Do not double the next dose.

STOPPING THE DRUG
If your doctor has advised you to take it, continue until directed to stop, even if you begin to feel better before the scheduled end of therapy. Otherwise, take as needed.

PROLONGED USE
Do not take cimetidine for more than 2 weeks unless told to do so by your doctor.

▼ PRECAUTIONS

Over 60: Adverse reactions may be more likely and more severe in older patients.

Driving and Hazardous Work: Do not drive or engage in hazardous work until you determine how the medicine affects you.

Alcohol: Avoid alcohol.

Pregnancy: Avoid or discontinue use if you are pregnant or trying to become pregnant.

Breast Feeding: Cimetidine passes into breast milk; avoid or discontinue use while breast feeding.

Infants and Children: Not recommended for use by children under age 16.

Special Concerns: Avoid cigarette smoking because it may increase stomach acid secretion and thus worsen the disease. Do not take cimetidine if you have ever had an allergic reaction to a histamine (H2) blocker. If stomach pain becomes worse while you are using the drug, tell your doctor right away.

OVERDOSE
Symptoms: No symptoms have been reported.

What to Do: An overdose is unlikely to be life-threatening. However, if someone takes a much larger dose than recommended, seek medical assistance right away.

▼ INTERACTIONS

DRUG INTERACTIONS
Consult your doctor for specific advice before using cimetidine if you are taking aminophylline, anticoagulants, caffeine, metoprolol, oxtriphylline, phenytoin, propranolol, theophylline, tricyclic antidepressants, itraconazole, ketoconazole, metronidazole.

FOOD INTERACTIONS
Carbonated drinks, citrus fruits and juices, caffeine-containing beverages, and other acidic foods or liquids may irritate the stomach or interfere with the therapeutic action of cimetidine.

DISEASE INTERACTIONS
Patients with kidney or liver disease or weakened immune systems should not use cimetidine or should use it in smaller, limited doses under careful medical supervision.

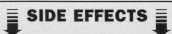

≡ SIDE EFFECTS ≡

SERIOUS
Irregular heart rhythm (palpitations), slowed heartbeat, severe blood problems resulting in unusual bleeding, bruising, fever, chills, and increased susceptibility to infection. Call your doctor immediately.

COMMON
Headache, fatigue, drowsiness, dizziness, nausea, vomiting, abdominal pain, diarrhea.

LESS COMMON
Blurred vision, decreased sexual desire or function, swelling of breasts in males or females, temporary hair loss, hallucinations, depression, insomnia, skin rash, hives, or redness.

CLEMASTINE FUMARATE

Available in: Tablets, syrup, extended-release tablets and caplets
Available as Generic? Yes
Drug Class: Antihistamine

▼ USAGE INFORMATION

WHY IT'S TAKEN
To prevent or relieve symptoms of hay fever and other allergies, and for itching skin and hives.

HOW IT WORKS
Clemastine blocks the effects of histamine, a naturally occurring substance within the body that causes swelling, itching, sneezing, watery eyes, hives, and other symptoms of allergic reactions.

▼ DOSAGE GUIDELINES

RANGE AND FREQUENCY
Adults and teenagers: 1.34 mg, 2 times a day (for hay fever), or 2.68 mg, 1 to 3 times a day (for hay fever or hives). Children ages 6 to 12: 0.67 mg (syrup) to 1.34 mg, 2 times a day.

ONSET OF EFFECT
15 minutes to 60 minutes.

DURATION OF ACTION
At least 12 hours.

DIETARY ADVICE
Take it with food, water, or milk to avoid stomach irritation. Drinking coffee or tea will help reduce drowsiness. Use sugarless gum, sugarless sour hard candy, or ice chips to ease dry mouth.

STORAGE
Store in a tightly sealed container away from heat and direct light.

MISSED DOSE
Take it as soon as you remember. If it is near the time for the next dose, skip the missed dose and resume your regular dosage schedule. Do not double the next dose.

STOPPING THE DRUG
You should take it as prescribed for the full treatment period, but you may stop if you are feeling better before the scheduled end of therapy. It may be taken as needed.

PROLONGED USE
No special problems are expected.

▼ PRECAUTIONS

Over 60: Adverse reactions may be more likely to occur and have greater severity in older patients.

≡ SIDE EFFECTS ≡

SERIOUS
Confusion, hallucinations, convulsions, blurred vision, difficulty urinating (urinary obstruction).

COMMON
Drowsiness; nausea; thickening of mucus; dry mouth, nose, and throat; dizziness; disturbed coordination.

LESS COMMON
Chills, headache, fatigue, vomiting, restlessness, irritability, nasal congestion, profuse sweating, diarrhea, constipation.

Driving and Hazardous Work: The use of clemastine may impair your ability to perform such tasks safely. Do not drive or engage in hazardous work until you know how the medicine is going to affect you.

Alcohol: Alcohol increases the likelihood and the severity of side effects like drowsiness and confusion.

Pregnancy: Animal studies with high doses of clemastine have found no birth defects. Human studies have not been done. Because the studies cannot rule out potential harm, the drug should be used during pregnancy only if it is clearly needed.

Breast Feeding: Clemastine passes into breast milk; do not use it while nursing.

Infants and Children: Children tend to be more sensitive to the effects of antihistamines. Symptoms of excitability, restlessness, and nightmares may occur.

OVERDOSE
Symptoms: Hallucinations, seizures, drowsiness, lethargy, coma.

What to Do: Call your doctor, emergency medical services (EMS), or the nearest poison control center immediately. A conscious patient should be induced to vomit using ipecac syrup.

▼ INTERACTIONS

DRUG INTERACTIONS
Sleeping pills, sedatives, tranquilizers, MAO inhibitors, and antidepressants can increase the sedative effects of clemastine. Anticholinergics may further increase the likelihood that drying of the mucous membranes and urinary obstruction will occur as side effects.

FOOD INTERACTIONS
No known food interactions.

DISEASE INTERACTIONS
Consult your doctor if you have any of the following: asthma, enlarged prostate, difficult urination, glaucoma, sleep apnea, or dry mouth or eyes.

CLOTRIMAZOLE

Available in: Topical cream, lotion, solution, oral lozenges, vaginal cream, tablets
Available as Generic? Yes
Drug Class: Antifungal

▼ USAGE INFORMATION

WHY IT'S TAKEN
To treat fungal infections of the mouth and throat (thrush), vaginal area (yeast infection), and the skin, such as tinea corporis (ringworm), tinea cruris (jock itch), tinea pedis (athlete's foot), and pityriasis versicolor ("sun fungus," a fungal skin condition that is characterized by fine scaly patches of varying shapes, sizes, and colors).

HOW IT WORKS
Clotrimazole prevents fungal organisms from producing vital substances required for growth and function.

▼ DOSAGE GUIDELINES

RANGE AND FREQUENCY
Topical cream, lotion, solution (for skin infections)—Adults and children: Apply twice a day, in the morning and in the evening. Oral lozenges (to treat thrush)—Adults and children age 5 and older: Dissolve one 10 mg lozenge in mouth 5 times a day for 14 days. To prevent thrush: Adults and children age 5 and older: Dissolve one 10 mg lozenge in mouth 3 times a day. Vaginal cream (for yeast infections)—Adults and teenagers: At bedtime, insert vaginally with an applicator 50 mg of 1% cream for 6 to 14 nights, or 100 mg of 2 % cream for 3 nights, or 500 mg of 10% cream for 1 night only. Vaginal tablets (for yeast infections)—Nonpregnant women and teenagers: At bedtime, insert one 100 mg tablet for 6 to 7 nights, or one 200 mg tablet for 3 nights, or one 500 mg tablet for 1 night only. Pregnant women and teenagers: At bedtime, insert one 100 mg tablet for 7 nights.

ONSET OF EFFECT
Unknown.

DURATION OF ACTION
Lozenges: 3 hours. Other forms: Unknown.

DIETARY ADVICE
No special restrictions.

STORAGE
Store in a tightly sealed container away from moisture, heat, and direct light. Do not allow it to freeze.

MISSED DOSE
Take it as soon as you remember. If it is near the time for the next dose, skip the missed dose and resume your regular dosage schedule. Do not double the next dose.

STOPPING THE DRUG
If you are using this drug by prescription, take it as prescribed for the full treatment period, even if you begin to feel better before the scheduled end of therapy. Recurrence of the infection is likely if you stop before the full treatment period is complete.

PROLONGED USE
Clotrimazole is generally prescribed for short-term therapy (1 to 14 days). Consult your doctor for further information.

▼ PRECAUTIONS

Over 60: No special problems are expected.

Driving and Hazardous Work: No special precautions are necessary.

Alcohol: No special precautions are necessary.

Pregnancy: Adequate studies on the use of clotrimazole during pregnancy have not been done; however, no problems have been reported. Consult your doctor for specific advice.

Breast Feeding: Clotrimazole may pass into breast milk; caution is advised. Consult your doctor for advice.

Infants and Children: Topical forms: No special warnings. Lozenges are not recommended for children younger than age 5. Vaginal forms: Not commonly prescribed for children under the age of 12.

Special Concerns: Do not chew or swallow lozenges. Clotrimazole lozenges may take 15 to 30 minutes to dissolve completely and are useless if swallowed.

OVERDOSE
Symptoms: An overdose with clotrimazole is unlikely.

What to Do: If someone should swallow a large amount of the medicine, call your doctor, emergency medical services (EMS), or the nearest poison control center immediately.

▼ INTERACTIONS

DRUG INTERACTIONS
No drug interactions have been reported.

FOOD INTERACTIONS
No food interactions have been reported.

DISEASE INTERACTIONS
No disease interactions have been reported.

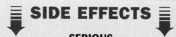

⬇ SIDE EFFECTS ⬇

SERIOUS
Topical: Hives, skin rash, itching, burning, peeling, stinging, redness, or other skin irritation not present prior to treatment. Lozenge and vaginal: None reported.

COMMON
Topical: None reported. Lozenge (when swallowed): Diarrhea, stomach cramping or pain, nausea or vomiting. Vaginal: Vaginal burning, itching, discharge, or other irritation not present prior to treatment.

LESS COMMON
Topical and lozenge: None reported. Vaginal: Headache, stomach cramps or pain, irritation or burning of sexual partner's penis.

COAL TAR

Available in: Cleansing bar, cream, gel, lotion, ointment, shampoo, liquid
Available as Generic? Yes
Drug Class: Antipsoriasis drug

▼ USAGE INFORMATION

WHY IT'S TAKEN
To treat skin conditions including dandruff, eczema, seborrheic dermatitis, and psoriasis.

HOW IT WORKS
Coal tar promotes softening, dissolution, and peeling of hard, scaly, roughened, or irregular surface skin. It also has antiseptic properties and fights fungal, bacterial, and parasitic organisms.

▼ DOSAGE GUIDELINES

RANGE AND FREQUENCY
Cleansing bar: Use 1 or 2 times a day as directed by your doctor. Cream: Apply to affected areas up to 4 times a day. Gel: Apply to affected areas 1 or 2 times a day. Lotion: Apply to affected areas as needed. Ointment: Apply to affected areas 2 or 3 times a day. Shampoo: Use once a day, once a week, or as directed by your doctor. Topical solution: Apply to skin or scalp or use in the bath, depending on product. Topical bath solution: Add appropriate amount to bath water; immerse yourself in the bath for 20 minutes. If you have

any questions about its use, consult your doctor.

ONSET OF EFFECT
Unknown.

DURATION OF ACTION
Unknown.

DIETARY ADVICE
Coal tar can be used without regard to diet.

STORAGE
Store in a tightly sealed container away from heat and direct light. Do not allow liquid forms to freeze.

MISSED DOSE
Apply it as soon as you remember. If it is near the time for the next dose, skip the missed dose and resume your regular dosage schedule. Do not apply a double dose.

STOPPING THE DRUG
If applying coal tar on medical order, the decision to stop using it should be made by your doctor. If you are using the drug on your own, you may stop treatment whenever you choose.

PROLONGED USE
Do not use coal tar for longer than the package specifies or your physician advises.

▼ PRECAUTIONS

Over 60: Coal tar is not expected to cause different side effects or problems in older patients than it does in younger persons.

Driving and Hazardous Work: The use of coal tar should not impair your ability to perform such tasks safely.

Alcohol: No special restrictions apply.

Pregnancy: Studies of coal tar use during pregnancy have not been done. Before you use coal tar, tell your doctor if you are pregnant or plan to become pregnant.

Breast Feeding: It is not known if coal tar passes into breast milk. Consult your doctor for specific advice.

Infants and Children: Use and dose in infants and children must be determined by your doctor.

Special Concerns: For external use only. Keep coal tar away from the eyes. If you accidentally get some of the medicine in your eyes, flush them thoroughly with water. After applying coal tar, protect the treated area from sunlight for 72 hours, and be sure to remove all coal tar before being exposed to sunlight or using a sunlamp. Do not apply coal tar to infected, blistered, raw, or oozing areas of the skin.

OVERDOSE
Symptoms: None reported.

What to Do: Emergency instructions not applicable.

Alphosyl, Aquatar, Balnetar Therapeutic Tar Bath, Cutar Water Dispersible Emollient Tar, Denorex Medicated Shampoo, DHS Tar Shampoo, Doak Oil Therapeutic Bath Treatment, Doctar Hair & Scalp Shampoo and Conditioner, Estar, Exorex, Fototar, Ionil T Plus, Lavatar, Medotar, Pentrax Anti-Dandruff Tar Shampoo, Psorigel, PsoriNail Topical Solution, T/Derm Tar Emollient, T/Gel Therapeutic Shampoo, Taraphilic, Tarbonis, Tarpaste 'Doak', Tegrin, Tersa-Tar Soapless Tar Shampoo, Theraplex T Shampoo, Zetar

▼ INTERACTIONS

DRUG INTERACTIONS
Consult your doctor for specific advice if you are using tetracyclines, psoralens, or retinoids. Also tell your doctor if you are using any other prescription or over-the-counter medication.

FOOD INTERACTIONS
No known food interactions.

DISEASE INTERACTIONS
You should not use coal tar if you have had a prior allergic reaction to it.

⬇ SIDE EFFECTS ⬇

SERIOUS
Skin irritation or rash not present before use of coal tar. Call your doctor immediately.

COMMON
Mild stinging, increased sensitivity to sunlight.

LESS COMMON
No less-common side effects have been reported.

CROMOLYN SODIUM INHALANT AND NASAL

Available in: Nasal solution
Available as Generic? Yes
Drug Class: Respiratory inhalant

▼ USAGE INFORMATION

WHY IT'S TAKEN
To control, through regular use, chronic bronchial asthma; or it may be used preventively just prior to exposure to certain conditions or substances (allergens such as pollen and dust mites, as well as cold air, chemicals, exercise, or air pollution) that can trigger an acute asthma attack (bronchospasm).

HOW IT WORKS
Cromolyn sodium inhibits the release of histamine, a naturally occurring substance that causes swelling, itching, sneezing, watery eyes, hives, and other symptoms of allergic reaction, including those that occur in association with an asthma attack.

▼ DOSAGE GUIDELINES

RANGE AND FREQUENCY
For hay fever: Adults and children age 6 and older: 1 spray in each nostril 3 to 6 times a day.

ONSET OF EFFECT
Unknown.

DURATION OF ACTION
Unknown.

DIETARY ADVICE
This medication should be taken 30 minutes before meals.

STORAGE
Store in a tightly sealed container away from heat and direct light.

MISSED DOSE
Take it as soon as you remember. If it is near the time for the next dose, skip the missed dose and resume your regular dosage schedule. Do not double the next dose.

STOPPING THE DRUG
The decision to stop taking cromolyn sodium should be made in consultation with your doctor.

PROLONGED USE
If your symptoms do not improve after 4 weeks, consult your doctor.

▼ PRECAUTIONS

Over 60: No special problems are expected in older patients.

Driving and Hazardous Work: No special problems are expected.

Alcohol: No special precautions are necessary.

Pregnancy: In studies done in animals, large doses of cromolyn sodium have caused a decrease in successful pregnancies and a decrease in fetal weight. Human studies have not yet been done. Before taking cromolyn sodium, tell your doctor if you are currently pregnant or if you plan to become pregnant.

Breast Feeding: It is not known whether cromolyn sodium passes into breast milk. Mothers who wish to breast feed while using this drug should discuss the matter with their doctor.

Infants and Children: The nasal form of cromolyn has not been studied in children. Consult your pediatrician for specific advice.

Special Concerns: Clean the inhaler and other devices at least once a week.

OVERDOSE
Symptoms: None reported.

What to Do: An overdose of cromolyn sodium is unlikely to be life-threatening. However, if someone takes a much larger dose than recommended, call your doctor, emergency medical services (EMS), or the nearest poison control center immediately.

▼ INTERACTIONS

DRUG INTERACTIONS
Before taking cromolyn sodium, check with your doctor if you are using any other prescription or over-the-counter drug.

FOOD INTERACTIONS
No known food interactions.

DISEASE INTERACTIONS
Before taking cromolyn sodium, consult your physician if you are undergoing treatment for any other medical condition.

☰ SIDE EFFECTS ☰

SERIOUS
Difficulty swallowing; hives; itching; swelling of face, lips, or eyelids; rash; nosebleeds. Call your doctor immediately.

COMMON
Inhalation: Throat irritation or dryness. Nasal: Increased sneezing; burning, stinging, or irritation in nose.

LESS COMMON
Nasal: Cough, headache, postnasal drip, unpleasant taste.

DEXTROMETHORPHAN

Available in: Capsules, lozenges, tablets, oral suspension, syrup
Available as Generic? Yes
Drug Class: Cough suppressant

▼ USAGE INFORMATION

WHY IT'S TAKEN
To relieve a dry or minimally productive cough (that is, a mild cough that rids the lungs of modest amounts of phlegm or mucus), commonly associated with allergies, colds, influenza, and certain lung disorders. This medicine is ideally useful when a mild or hacking cough would interrupt sleep or interfere with your daily activities.

HOW IT WORKS
Dextromethorphan works by directly reducing the sensitivity of the cough center—the part of the brain that responds to stimuli in the lower respiratory passages that irritate and trigger the cough reflex.

▼ DOSAGE GUIDELINES

RANGE AND FREQUENCY
Adults: 10 to 20 mg every 4 hours or 30 mg every 6 to 8 hours; 30 to 60 mg of extended-release liquid twice a day. Children 6 to 12: 5 to 10 mg every 4 hours or 30 mg of extended-release liquid twice a day. Children 2 to 6: 2.5 to 5 mg every 4 hours, or 7.5 mg every 6 to 8 hours, or 15 mg of the extended-release liquid twice a day. Children under 2: Dosage must be individualized.

ONSET OF EFFECT
15 to 30 minutes.

DURATION OF ACTION
Up to 6 hours.

DIETARY ADVICE
No special restrictions.

STORAGE
Store in a tightly sealed container away from heat, moisture, and direct light.

MISSED DOSE
Take it as soon as you remember. However, if it is near the time for the next dose, skip the missed dose and resume your regular dosage schedule. Do not double the next dose.

STOPPING THE DRUG
Take it as prescribed for the full treatment period. However, you may stop taking the drug if you are feeling better before the scheduled end of therapy. If the cough does not improve after 7 days, consult your doctor.

PROLONGED USE
No problems are expected.

▼ PRECAUTIONS

Over 60: Side effects may be more frequent and severe than in younger persons. Smaller doses for shorter periods may be needed. If this drug is used to control coughing, other treatment measures may be needed to liquefy any accumulation of thick mucus that may form in the bronchial tubes.

Driving and Hazardous Work: Determine whether it causes drowsiness or dizziness before you drive or engage in hazardous work.

Alcohol: Avoid alcohol while using this drug; it may increase the risk of sedation.

Pregnancy: Ask your doctor whether the benefits of the drug justify the possible risk to the fetus.

Breast Feeding: Dextromethorphan may pass into breast milk; caution is advised. Consult your doctor for specific advice about taking dextromethorphan while you are nursing.

Infants and Children: Doses for children under 2 must be individualized; consult your pediatrician.

Special Concerns: Do not take dextromethorphan to relieve a cough that is caused by asthma, emphysema, or smoking.

OVERDOSE
Symptoms: Nausea, vomiting, nervousness and agitation, extreme drowsiness or dizziness, extreme irritability or mood changes, hallucinations, blurred vision, uncontrollable eye movement, inability to urinate, confusion, loss of consciousness, or coma.

What to Do: Call your doctor, emergency medical services (EMS), or the nearest poison control center immediately.

▼ INTERACTIONS

DRUG INTERACTIONS
Taking it with a sedative or other depressant can increase the sedative effects of both drugs. Using doxepin increases the toxic effects of both drugs. Taking an MAO inhibitor can cause a high fever, disorientation, or loss of consciousness. Using quinidine increases the risk of experiencing side effects with dextromethorphan.

FOOD INTERACTIONS
No known food interactions.

DISEASE INTERACTIONS
Caution is advised when taking dextromethorphan. Consult your doctor before taking this drug if you have a history of asthma or impaired liver function.

≡ SIDE EFFECTS ≡

SERIOUS
Serious side effects occur only in cases of overdose (see Overdose).

COMMON
No common side effects are associated with this drug.

LESS COMMON
Mild dizziness or sedation, nausea or vomiting, abdominal pain. Such symptoms are more likely to occur at the beginning of therapy and tend to diminish as your body becomes accustomed to taking the drug. Consult your doctor if they persist or interfere with daily activities.

DIMENHYDRINATE

Available in: Capsules, tablets, elixir, syrup
Available as Generic? Yes
Drug Class: Antihistamine

▼ USAGE INFORMATION

WHY IT'S TAKEN
To relieve nausea and vomiting and to treat or prevent motion sickness.

HOW IT WORKS
Dimenhydrinate directly inhibits the stimulation of certain nerves in the brain and inner ear to suppress nausea, vomiting, dizziness, and vertigo.

▼ DOSAGE GUIDELINES

RANGE AND FREQUENCY
Adults: 50 to 100 mg every 4 to 6 hours. Children ages 6 to 12: 25 to 50 mg every 6 to 8 hours. Children ages 2 to 6: 12.5 to 25 mg every 6 to 8 hours. To prevent motion sickness, take this drug at least 30 minutes, and preferably 1 to 2 hours, before you are planning to travel.

ONSET OF EFFECT
Within 20 to 30 minutes.

DURATION OF ACTION
3 to 6 hours.

DIETARY ADVICE
This drug can be taken with food or milk to minimize any gastrointestinal distress from occurring.

STORAGE
Store in a tightly sealed container in a dry place away from heat and direct light.

MISSED DOSE
Take it as soon as you remember. However, if it is near the time for the next dose, skip the missed dose and resume your regular dosage schedule. Do not double the next dose.

STOPPING THE DRUG
You should take it according to package directions for the full treatment period, but you may stop if you are feeling better before the scheduled end of therapy.

PROLONGED USE
Take this drug only as long as it is needed.

▼ PRECAUTIONS

Over 60: Older persons are more sensitive to the effects of dimenhydrinate. Dizziness, drowsiness, confusion, difficult or painful urination, and other side effects are more likely to occur.

Driving and Hazardous Work: Do not drive or engage in hazardous work until you determine how the medicine affects you.

Alcohol: Avoid alcohol.

Pregnancy: Animal studies with high doses of dimenhydrinate have found no birth defects. Human studies have not been done. Because the studies cannot rule out harm, the drug should be used during pregnancy only if it is clearly needed.

Breast Feeding: Dimenhydrinate may pass into breast milk; caution is advised; avoid or discontinue use while breast feeding.

Infants and Children: The safety and efficacy of this drug in children under 2 years of age (age 6 for the suppository form) have not been established. Older children are especially sensitive to the drug's side effects.

Special Concerns: Children should be observed carefully for signs of side effects; they are more likely to develop serious complications from these medications, and younger children are often unable to describe changes in the way that they are feeling.

OVERDOSE
Symptoms: Seizures, hallucinations, drowsiness, difficulty breathing, unconsciousness.

What to Do: An overdose of dimenhydrinate is unlikely to be life-threatening. However, if someone takes a much larger dose than recommended, call your doctor, emergency medical services (EMS), or the nearest poison control center immediately.

▼ INTERACTIONS

DRUG INTERACTIONS
Consult your doctor for specific advice if you are taking any narcotic pain relievers, sedatives, tranquilizers, antidepressants, antibiotics, aspirin, barbiturates, cisplatin, diuretics, or theophylline.

FOOD INTERACTIONS
No known food interactions.

DISEASE INTERACTIONS
Caution is advised when taking dimenhydrinate. Consult your doctor if you have glaucoma or an enlarged prostate.

≡ SIDE EFFECTS ≡

SERIOUS
No serious side effects are associated with this drug.

COMMON
Drowsiness.

LESS COMMON
Headache, blurred vision, palpitations, loss of coordination, dry mouth, low blood pressure causing dizziness and weakness, ringing in ears.

DIPHENHYDRAMINE HYDROCHLORIDE

Available in: Capsules, elixir, syrup, tablets
Available as Generic? Yes
Drug Class: Antihistamine

▼ USAGE INFORMATION

WHY IT'S TAKEN
To relieve hay fever symptoms, itching skin and hives, motion sickness, nonproductive cough due to cold or hay fever, and sleeping difficulty; also used to treat symptoms of Parkinson's disease.

HOW IT WORKS
It blocks the effects of histamine, a naturally occurring substance that causes swelling, itching, sneezing, and watery eyes. In patients with Parkinson's disease, it decreases tremors and muscle stiffness.

▼ DOSAGE GUIDELINES

RANGE AND FREQUENCY
For hay fever symptoms—Capsules, elixir, syrup, tablets: Adults and teenagers: 25 to 50 mg every 4 to 6 hours. Children younger than age 6: 6.25 to 12.5 mg every 4 to 6 hours. Children ages 6 to 12: 12.5 to 25 mg every 4 to 6 hours. For nausea, vomiting and dizziness—Capsules, elixir, syrup, tablets: Adults: 25 to 50 mg every 4 to 6 hours. Children: 1 to 1.5 mg per 2.2 lbs every 4 to 6 hours. For Parkinson's disease—Capsules, elixir, syrup, tablets: Adults: 25 mg, 3 times a day. Doctor may gradually increase dose. As a sedative—Capsules, elixir, syrup, tablets: Adults: 50 mg 20 to 30 minutes before bedtime. For cough—Liquid: Adults and teenagers: 25 mg every 4 to 6 hours. Children ages 2 to 6: 6.25 mg (½ teaspoon) every 4 to 6 hours. Children ages 6 to 12: 12.5 mg (1 teaspoon) every 4 to 6 hours.

ONSET OF EFFECT
Capsules, elixir, syrup, or tablets: 15 minutes.

DURATION OF ACTION
6 to 8 hours.

DIETARY ADVICE
Take diphenhydramine with food or milk to reduce gastrointestinal distress, a possible side effect.

STORAGE
Store in a dry place away from heat and direct light. Prevent liquid forms from freezing.

MISSED DOSE
Take it as soon as you remember. If it is near the time for the next dose, skip the missed dose and resume your regular dosage schedule. Do not double the next dose.

STOPPING THE DRUG
Stop taking this drug and call your doctor if it is not effective after 5 days.

PROLONGED USE
No special problems have been reported.

▼ PRECAUTIONS

Over 60: Adverse reactions may be more likely and more severe.

Driving and Hazardous Work: Do not drive or engage in hazardous work until you determine how the medicine affects you. Use of this drug is a disqualification for piloting aircraft.

Alcohol: Alcohol may increase the likelihood and severity of side effects such as drowsiness and mental confusion.

Pregnancy: No birth defects have been reported in animals. Studies of pregnant women have found no significant increase in birth defects.

Breast Feeding: Diphenhydramine passes into breast milk; avoid or discontinue use while nursing.

Infants and Children: This drug is not recommended for children under the age of 2.

Special Concerns: Children should be observed carefully for signs of side effects; they are more likely to develop serious complications, and younger children are often unable to describe changes in the way that they are feeling.

OVERDOSE
Symptoms: Marked drowsiness, dilated and unreactive pupils, fever, excitability, breathing interruptions, combativeness, mental confusion, loss of coordination, weak pulse, seizures, and loss of consciousness.

What to Do: Call your doctor, emergency medical services (EMS), or the nearest poison control center immediately.

▼ INTERACTIONS

DRUG INTERACTIONS
Consult your doctor for specific advice before using diphenhydramine if you are also taking anticholinergics, alcohol, disopyramide, central nervous system depressants, or MAO inhibitors.

FOOD INTERACTIONS
No known food interactions.

DISEASE INTERACTIONS
Consult your doctor if you have a history of severe respiratory disease, glaucoma, urinary obstruction, or prostate enlargement.

≡ SIDE EFFECTS ≡

SERIOUS
No serious side effects are associated with this drug.

COMMON
Drowsiness, dry mouth, nausea, thickening of mucus.

LESS COMMON
Confusion, difficult urination, blurred vision.

DOCUSATE

Available in: Capsules, tablets, liquid, syrup
Available as Generic? Yes
Drug Class: Stool softener

▼ USAGE INFORMATION

WHY IT'S TAKEN
To prevent constipation (but not to treat existing constipation). Recommended for persons who should not strain during defecation, such as those recovering from rectal or heart surgery, or women who experience constipation after childbirth.

HOW IT WORKS
Docusate draws liquid into stools, forming a softer mass.

▼ DOSAGE GUIDELINES

RANGE AND FREQUENCY
Adults and teenagers: 50 to 500 mg once a day until bowel movements return to normal. Children ages 6 to 12: 40 to 140 mg once a day. Liquid forms should be mixed with milk or fruit juice.

ONSET OF EFFECT
Within 24 to 72 hours.

DURATION OF ACTION
Up to 72 hours.

DIETARY ADVICE
Add high-fiber foods like bran and fresh fruits and vegetables to your diet. Drink at least 6 glasses (8 oz each) of water or other liquids a day to help soften stools.

STORAGE
Store in a tightly sealed container kept away from heat, moisture, and direct light.

MISSED DOSE
Take it as soon as you remember. If it is near the time for the next dose, skip the missed dose and resume your regular dosage schedule. Do not double the next dose.

STOPPING THE DRUG
Take it as advised for the full treatment period. However, you may stop taking the drug if you are feeling better and normal bowel function has returned before the scheduled end of therapy.

PROLONGED USE
Docusate should not be taken for more than 1 week unless you are under your doctor's supervision. Be aware that overuse can make you dependent on it and may cause damage to the nerves, muscles, and other tissues of the bowel and lead to vitamin and mineral deficiency.

▼ PRECAUTIONS

Over 60: No special problems are expected.

Driving and Hazardous Work: The use of docusate should not impair your ability to perform such tasks safely.

Alcohol: No special precautions are necessary.

Pregnancy: Before taking docusate, tell your doctor if you are pregnant or plan to become pregnant.

Breast Feeding: No special problems are expected if you take docusate while nursing.

Infants and Children: Do not give docusate to children under age 6 unless it is prescribed by your doctor.

Special Concerns: Do not take mineral oil while you are taking docusate.

OVERDOSE
Symptoms: Weakness, sweating, muscle cramps, irregular heartbeat.

What to Do: An overdose of docusate is unlikely to be life-threatening. However, if someone takes a much larger dose than prescribed, call your doctor, emergency medical services (EMS), or the nearest poison control center immediately.

▼ INTERACTIONS

DRUG INTERACTIONS
A number of drugs may interact with docusate if they are ingested at or near the time it is taken. Consult your doctor for specific advice if you are taking any other oral drug within 2 hours before or after taking docusate.

FOOD INTERACTIONS
No known food interactions.

DISEASE INTERACTIONS
This drug cannot be used by people with intestinal obstruction or appendicitis. The symptoms of these conditions include vomiting, abdominal rigidity and tenderness, and fever. Call your doctor or emergency medical services (EMS) immediately if you suspect you may be suffering from intestinal obstruction or appendicitis.

▼ SIDE EFFECTS

SERIOUS
Severe cramping. Stop taking the drug and call your doctor immediately.

COMMON
Diarrhea, mild abdominal cramps.

LESS COMMON
Throat irritation, laxative dependence. Consult your doctor if you cannot maintain normal bowel habits without docusate for more than 2 weeks.

EPHEDRINE

Available in: Capsules
Available as Generic? Yes
Drug Class: Adrenergic bronchodilator

▼ USAGE INFORMATION

WHY IT'S TAKEN
To relieve bronchial asthma, to decrease nasal and lower respiratory congestion, and to suppress allergic reactions. Ephedrine commonly appears in combination with other medications.

HOW IT WORKS
Ephedrine prevents cells from releasing histamine, a naturally occurring substance that causes swelling, itching, sneezing, watery eyes, hives, and other symptoms of allergic reaction. It also relaxes the smooth muscle surrounding the bronchial tubes, widening the airways, and causes constriction of blood vessels in the nose, which helps to open the nasal passages.

▼ DOSAGE GUIDELINES

RANGE AND FREQUENCY
Adults: 25 to 50 mg every 3 or 4 hours, if needed. Children: 3 mg per 2.2 lbs (1 kg) of body weight per day, in 4 to 6 divided doses.

ONSET OF EFFECT
15 to 60 minutes.

DURATION OF ACTION
3 to 5 hours.

DIETARY ADVICE
Swallow capsules with water and drink plenty of fluids.

STORAGE
Store in a dry place in a tightly sealed container away from heat and direct light.

MISSED DOSE
Take it if you remember within 2 hours. If not, skip the missed dose and resume your normal dosage schedule. Do not double the next dose.

STOPPING THE DRUG
You may stop taking this drug at your own discretion. Consult your doctor.

PROLONGED USE
This drug may lose its effectiveness if taken steadily for 3 to 4 days. Men with an enlarged prostate gland may have difficulty urinating.

▼ PRECAUTIONS

Over 60: Adverse reactions may be more likely and more severe. Small doses are advisable until individual response has been evaluated.

Driving and Hazardous Work: Ephedrine may cause dizziness. Do not drive or engage in hazardous work until you determine how it affects you.

Alcohol: No special precautions are necessary.

Pregnancy: Consult your doctor; benefits must clearly outweigh risks.

Breast Feeding: Ephedrine passes into breast milk and may be harmful to the child; do not use it while nursing.

Infants and Children: Use caution. Ask your doctor if the benefits of ephedrine justify possible risk to the child.

Special Concerns: Ephedrine can cause insomnia. Take the last dose at least 2 hours before bedtime. Before you take ephedrine, tell your doctor if you will have surgery requiring general anesthesia, including dental surgery, within 2 months.

OVERDOSE
Symptoms: Severe anxiety, convulsions, coma, breathing difficulty, confusion, delirium, rapid and irregular pulse, muscle tremors.

What to Do: Call your doctor, emergency medical services (EMS), or the nearest poison control center immediately.

▼ INTERACTIONS

DRUG INTERACTIONS
Consult your doctor for specific advice if you are taking tricyclic antidepressants, high blood pressure medication, beta-blockers, dextrothyroxine, digitalis drugs, ergot-containing preparations, furazolidone, guanadrel, guanethidine, heart medication, methyldopa, MAO inhibitors, nitrates, phenothiazines, pseudoephedrine, rauwolfia alkaloids, sympathomimetic drugs, terazosin, theophylline, or any nonprescription drug for a cough, cold, allergy, or asthma.

FOOD INTERACTIONS
No known food interactions.

DISEASE INTERACTIONS
Caution is advised when taking ephedrine. Consult your doctor if you have any of the following: enlarged prostate, high blood pressure, history of seizures, diabetes, an overactive thyroid gland, or Parkinson's disease.

≡ SIDE EFFECTS ≡

SERIOUS
Irregular heartbeats; hallucinations with high doses; shortness of breath. Call your doctor.

COMMON
Nervousness, rapid heartbeat, paleness, insomnia.

LESS COMMON
Dizziness, loss of appetite, nausea, vomiting, muscle cramps, headache, difficult or painful urination.

EPINEPHRINE HYDROCHLORIDE

Available in: Inhalation aerosols and solutions, eye drops
Available as Generic? Yes
Drug Class: Bronchodilator/sympathomimetic; antiglaucoma agent

▼ USAGE INFORMATION

WHY IT'S TAKEN
To treat bronchial asthma, emphysema, and other lung diseases. Epinephrine is also a primary treatment for anaphylaxis; that is, hypersensitive (allergic) reaction to drugs or other substances. It may also be used to treat nasal congestion, to prolong the action of anesthetics, and to treat cardiac arrest. The ophthalmic form of the drug is used to treat glaucoma.

HOW IT WORKS
Epinephrine widens constricted airways in the lungs by relaxing smooth muscles that surround bronchial passages. It also raises blood pressure by constricting small blood vessels, increases the heart rate and strength of heart contractions, and decreases fluid pressure in the eye.

▼ DOSAGE GUIDELINES

RANGE AND FREQUENCY
It may be used when needed to relieve breathing difficulty. For adults and children 4 years of age or older with asthma—Inhaled aerosol: 200 micrograms (mcg) to 275 mcg (1 puff), repeated if needed after 1 or 2 minutes, with doses taken at least 3 hours apart. Inhalation solution: 1 puff of 1% solution repeated after 1 or 2 minutes, if needed. For open-angle glaucoma—1 or 2 drops of 1% or 2% solution, once or twice daily.

ONSET OF EFFECT
Within 5 minutes.

DURATION OF ACTION
1 to 3 hours.

DIETARY ADVICE
No special concerns.

STORAGE
Store in a tightly sealed container, away from moisture, heat, and direct light.

MISSED DOSE
Take your missed dose as soon as you remember, unless the time for your next scheduled dose is within the next 2 hours, in which case skip the missed dose. Take your next scheduled dose at the proper time and resume your regular dosage schedule. Do not take a double dose.

STOPPING THE DRUG
Take the drug exactly as prescribed. Contact your doctor if you do not respond to the strength of the dosage you have been given.

PROLONGED USE
Tolerance to epinephrine may develop with prolonged use.

▼ PRECAUTIONS

Over 60: Adverse reactions may be more likely and more severe in older patients.

Driving and Hazardous Work: Do not drive or engage in hazardous work until you determine how the medicine affects you.

Alcohol: It may increase the excretion of epinephrine in the urine.

Pregnancy: Benefits of taking the drug must outweigh the potential risks; consult your doctor for specific advice.

Breast Feeding: Epinephrine passes into the breast milk. Consult your doctor for specific advice.

Infants and Children: They may be especially sensitive to epinephrine; fainting by children with asthma taking the drug has been reported.

Special Concerns: Do not use without a prescription, unless your problem has been diagnosed as asthma. Take aerosol doses exactly as directed; overuse has caused sudden death.

OVERDOSE

Symptoms: Chest discomfort, chills or fever, dizziness, seizures, irregular heartbeat, trouble breathing.

What to Do: Call your doctor, emergency medical services (EMS), or the nearest poison control center immediately.

▼ INTERACTIONS

DRUG INTERACTIONS
Consult your doctor for specific advice if you are taking anesthetics, tricyclic antidepressants, antidiabetic agents, antihypertensives or diuretics, beta-blockers, digitalis drugs, ergoloid mesylates, maprotiline, ergotamine, or MAO inhibitors.

FOOD INTERACTIONS
Avoid any foods that have previously triggered an allergic reaction or asthma attack.

DISEASE INTERACTIONS
The benefits of taking the drug need to be weighed against the potential risks if you have any of the following conditions: organic brain damage, diabetes mellitus, Parkinson's disease, heart or blood vessel disease, or overactive thyroid.

≣ SIDE EFFECTS ≣

▼ SERIOUS ▼
Bluish color of skin, severe dizziness, flushing, and difficulty breathing may indicate an allergic reaction to sulfites in the medication. Contact your doctor immediately.

COMMON
Dry mouth and throat; trembling; headaches. Check with your doctor if these symptoms continue or become bothersome.

LESS COMMON
Eye pain or headache from using eye drops.

FAMOTIDINE

Available in: Tablets, powder for suspension, orally disintegrating and chewable tablets
Available as Generic? No
Drug Class: Histamine (H2) blocker

▼ USAGE INFORMATION

WHY IT'S TAKEN
To treat heartburn, ulcers of the stomach and duodenum, conditions that cause excess production of stomach acid (such as Zollinger-Ellison syndrome), and gastroesophageal reflux (backwash of stomach acid into the esophagus, resulting in heartburn). The chewable tablets are taken for prevention or treatment of heartburn.

HOW IT WORKS
Famotidine blocks the action of histamine (a compound that is produced in the body's cells), which in turn decreases the stomach's secretion of hydrochloric acid. Once the production of stomach acid is decreased, the body is better able to heal itself.

▼ DOSAGE GUIDELINES

RANGE AND FREQUENCY
To prevent heartburn: 10 mg, 1 hour before meals. For excess stomach acid: 20 to 160 mg every 6 hours. For acid reflux disease: 20 mg twice a day for up to 6 weeks. For stomach ulcers: 40 mg once a day for 8 weeks. For duodenal ulcers: To start, 40 mg once a day at bedtime or 20 mg twice a day; later, 20 mg once a day. Chewable tablets—For treatment of heartburn: Chew one tablet. For prevention of heartburn: Chew one tablet 15 to 60 minutes before eating.

ONSET OF EFFECT
The nonprescription form may take 45 minutes to relieve heartburn.

DURATION OF ACTION
Up to 12 hours.

DIETARY ADVICE
Take it after meals or with milk to minimize stomach irritation. Avoid foods that cause stomach irritation. Take chewable tablet with a glass of water.

STORAGE
Store tablets in a tightly sealed container away from heat, moisture, and direct light. After powder vials are reconstituted, store the medicine in the refrigerator, but keep it from freezing. Discard after 30 days.

MISSED DOSE
Take it as soon as you remember. If it is near the time for the next dose, skip the missed dose and resume your regular dosage schedule. Do not double the next dose.

STOPPING THE DRUG
If your doctor advises you to take it, do not stop without consulting him or her.

PROLONGED USE
Do not take the prescription drug for more than 8 weeks unless your doctor orders it. Do not take the over-the-counter drug for more than 2 weeks unless otherwise instructed by your doctor.

▼ PRECAUTIONS

Over 60: Adverse reactions may be more likely and more severe in older patients.

Driving and Hazardous Work: Do not drive or engage in hazardous work until you determine how the medicine affects you.

Alcohol: Avoid alcohol while taking this drug; it may slow recovery. Also, this drug increases blood alcohol levels.

Pregnancy: Risks vary, depending on patient and dosage. Consult your physician for advice.

Breast Feeding: Famotidine passes into breast milk; you should avoid or discontinue use while breast feeding.

Infants and Children: Famotidine is rarely recommended for infants and children.

Special Concerns: If necessary, famotidine may be given with antacids. Avoid cigarette smoking because it may increase secretion of stomach acid and thus worsen the disease.

OVERDOSE
Symptoms: Confusion, slurred speech, rapid heartbeat, difficulty breathing, delirium.

What to Do: Call your doctor, emergency medical services (EMS), or the nearest poison control center immediately.

▼ INTERACTIONS

DRUG INTERACTIONS
None reported.

FOOD INTERACTIONS
Carbonated drinks, citrus fruits and juices, caffeine-containing beverages, and other acidic foods or liquids may irritate the stomach or interfere with the therapeutic action of famotidine.

DISEASE INTERACTIONS
Patients with kidney disease should use famotidine in smaller, limited doses under careful supervision by a physician.

≡ SIDE EFFECTS ≡

SERIOUS
Irregular heart rhythm (palpitations), slowed heartbeat, severe blood problems resulting in unusual bleeding, bruising, fever, chills, and increased susceptibility to infection. Call your doctor immediately.

COMMON
Headache, fatigue, drowsiness, dizziness, nausea, vomiting, abdominal pain, diarrhea, constipation.

LESS COMMON
Blurred vision, decreased sexual desire or function, temporary hair loss, hallucinations, depression, insomnia, skin rash, hives, or redness.

FERROUS SALTS

Available in: Capsules, drops, elixir, solution, tablets
Available as Generic? Yes
Drug Class: Dietary supplement

▼ USAGE INFORMATION

WHY IT'S TAKEN
To help increase the body's stores of iron, a mineral essential to the manufacture of red blood cells. An insufficient number of red blood cells results in anemia.

HOW IT WORKS
Ferrous salts are required for the production of hemoglobin in developing red blood cells. Hemoglobin is a complex iron-based protein in the red cell that carries oxygen to the body's tissues and carries carbon dioxide gas away from the tissues to be exhaled by the lungs.

▼ DOSAGE GUIDELINES

RANGE AND FREQUENCY
For iron deficiency, 325 mg, 3 times a day. Children: 5 to 10 mg for every 2.2 lbs (1 kg) of body weight 3 times a day.

ONSET OF EFFECT
From 5 to 7 days. Depending on the extent of the deficiency, more than 3 months of therapy may be needed for maximum benefit to be realized.

DURATION OF ACTION
Depends on the body's ability to utilize it.

DIETARY ADVICE
Take 1 hour before or 2 hours after eating.

STORAGE
Store in a tightly sealed container away from heat and direct light. Keep the liquid form from freezing.

MISSED DOSE
Take it as soon as you remember. If it is near the time for the next dose, skip the missed dose and resume your regular dosage schedule. Do not double the next dose.

STOPPING THE DRUG
If the medication was prescribed, the decision to stop taking this supplement should be made by your doctor.

PROLONGED USE
Prolonged use may result in the accumulation of iron in the tissues, the effects of which can include liver damage, heart problems, diabetes, erectile dysfunction, and unusually bronzed skin. Do not take iron supplements without consulting your doctor.

▼ PRECAUTIONS

Over 60: Problems in older adults have not been reported with intake of normal daily recommended amounts.

Driving and Hazardous Work: No problems expected.

Alcohol: Avoid alcohol while taking this medication because it may cause excess absorption of iron.

Pregnancy: This medication should be taken during pregnancy only if your doctor so advises.

Breast Feeding: No problems are expected during breast feeding; however, consult your doctor before taking ferrous salts.

Infants and Children: No unusual problems reported in infants and children. Close medical supervision is nonetheless recommended, and iron tablets should be stored out of reach of small children to avoid accidental ingestion, which can be severely toxic.

Special Concerns: The genetic disorder called hemochromatosis, in which the body accumulates excessive iron, is very common. Iron deficiency may also be the first indication of a gastrointestinal malignancy. Therefore, iron should only be used on the advice of a physician. Liquid forms of iron can stain the teeth. To prevent stains, mix each dose in water, fruit juice, or tomato juice and drink it through a straw. When using a dropper, place the dose on the back of the tongue and drink a glass of water or juice. Tooth stains can be removed by brushing with baking soda or 3% hydrogen peroxide.

OVERDOSE
Symptoms: Lethargy, nausea, vomiting, weak and rapid pulse, dehydration, loss of consciousness.

What to Do: Call your doctor, emergency medical services (EMS), or the nearest poison control center immediately.

▼ INTERACTIONS

DRUG INTERACTIONS
The following drugs may interact with ferrous salts and prevent their absorption: antacids, antibiotics, fluoroquinolones, levodopa, cholestyramine, or vitamin E. Consult your doctor for specific advice.

FOOD INTERACTIONS
Some foods can reduce the effect of this drug. The following foods should be avoided or taken in small amounts for at least 1 hour before and 2 hours after iron is taken: Eggs, milk, spinach, cheese, yogurt, tea, coffee, whole-grain bread, cereal, and bran.

DISEASE INTERACTIONS
Consult your doctor if you have any of the following: a history of alcoholism; kidney disease; liver disease; porphyria; rheumatoid arthritis; asthma; allergies; heart disease; or a stomach ulcer, colitis, or another intestinal problem.

≣ SIDE EFFECTS ≣

SERIOUS
No serious side effects are associated with ferrous salts, except for iron overload due to prolonged, inappropriate use of the mineral.

COMMON
Nausea, constipation, black stools.

LESS COMMON
Stained teeth (with liquid forms), stomach pain, vomiting, diarrhea.

FOLIC ACID (FOLACIN; FOLATE)

Available in: Tablets
Available as Generic? Yes
Drug Class: Vitamin

▼ USAGE INFORMATION

WHY IT'S TAKEN
The vitamin folic acid (also known as folacin and folate) is prescribed for treatment or prevention of certain types of anemia that result from folic acid deficiency. Such deficiencies may occur due to insufficient intake of folic acid (a result of poor diet or malnutrition), an inability to absorb the vitamin (as occurs in gastrointestinal disease), impaired ability to utilize the vitamin (due to excessive alcohol intake or the use of the anticonvulsant drug phenytoin), or as a result of conditions requiring increased amounts of folic acid (as occurs with pregnancy, breast feeding, hemodialysis, hemolytic anemia, and bone marrow failure).

HOW IT WORKS
Folic acid enhances chemical reactions within the body that contribute to the production of red blood cells, the manufacture of DNA needed for cell replication, and the metabolism of amino acids (compounds necessary for the manufacture of proteins).

▼ DOSAGE GUIDELINES

RANGE AND FREQUENCY
For severe deficiency—Adults and children, regardless of age: 1 mg daily. For daily supplementation following correction of severe deficiency—Adults and adolescents: 1 mg, once daily. During pregnancy: 400 micrograms (mcg), once daily. While breast feeding: 260 to 280 mcg, once daily. Children, newborn to 3 years of age: 25 to 50 mcg, once daily; child 4 to 6 years of age: 75 mcg, once daily; child 7 to 10 years of age: 100 mcg, once daily.

ONSET OF EFFECT
Folic acid is used immediately by the body for a number of vital chemical functions.

DURATION OF ACTION
Folic acid is required by your body on a daily basis throughout a lifetime.

DIETARY ADVICE
Maintain your usual food and fluid intake. Increase fluids if you have a fever or diarrhea, in hot weather, or during exercise. Follow your doctor's dietary advice (such as low-fat, low-salt, or low-cholesterol restrictions) to improve control over high blood pressure and heart disease.

STORAGE
Store in a tightly sealed container away from heat and direct light. Keep away from moisture and extremes in temperature.

MISSED DOSE
Take it as soon as you remember. If it is near the time for the next dose, skip the missed dose and resume your regular dosage schedule. Do not double the next dose.

STOPPING THE DRUG
The decision to stop taking the drug should be made by your doctor.

PROLONGED USE
Therapy with folacin may require weeks or months.

▼ PRECAUTIONS

Over 60: No special problems are expected in older patients.

Driving and Hazardous Work: The use of folic acid should not impair your ability to perform such tasks safely.

Alcohol: Alcohol impairs the body's utilization of folic acid; avoid it completely if you are taking folic acid.

Pregnancy: Folic acid supplementation is recommended during pregnancy.

Breast Feeding: Folic acid supplementation is recommended while nursing.

Infants and Children: Folic acid may be used regardless of age.

Special Concerns: Folic acid ingestion can mask vitamin B12 deficiency and lead to irreversible neurological damage; therefore, folic acid should be taken only upon the recommendation of your doctor. Folic acid deficiency should not occur and supplementation is not necessary in healthy individuals who consume a normal balanced diet.

OVERDOSE
Symptoms: No specific ones have been reported.

What to Do: An overdose of folic acid is not life-threatening. No emergency procedures are warranted.

▼ INTERACTIONS

DRUG INTERACTIONS
Consult your doctor for advice if you are taking pain relievers, antibiotics, anticonvulsants, epoetin, estrogens, oral contraceptives, methotrexate, pyrimethamine, triamterene, sulfasalazine, or zinc supplements.

FOOD INTERACTIONS
No known food interactions.

DISEASE INTERACTIONS
Consult your doctor if you have pernicious anemia.

≣ SIDE EFFECTS ≣

SERIOUS
Wheezing, breathing difficulty, chest pain, swelling, tightness in throat or chest, dizziness, rash, itching. Such symptoms may indicate a serious allergic reaction, although this is extremely rare.

COMMON
The are no known common side effects associated with the use of folic acid.

LESS COMMON
Mild allergic reactions.

GLYCERIN RECTAL

Available in: Rectal solution, rectal suppositories
Available as Generic? Yes
Drug Class: Hyperosmotic laxative

▼ USAGE INFORMATION

WHY IT'S TAKEN
To treat constipation.

HOW IT WORKS
Glycerin attracts and retains water in the intestine, softening stools and inducing the urge to defecate.

▼ DOSAGE GUIDELINES

RANGE AND FREQUENCY
Adults and children age 6 and older: Insert one suppository or 5 to 15 ml of solution as rectal enema and retain for 15 minutes. Do not lubricate suppositories with anything other than water.

ONSET OF EFFECT
Within 15 to 60 minutes.

DURATION OF ACTION
Only while the solution or suppository is within the rectum.

DIETARY ADVICE
Maintain your usual food and fluid intake. Increase your intake of fluids if you have a fever or diarrhea, during hot weather, or during exercise.

STORAGE
Store solutions and suppositories away from moisture, heat, and direct light. While suppositories may be refrigerated, do not allow them to freeze.

MISSED DOSE
Laxatives are usually prescribed for use only on an as-needed basis and are not meant to be taken regularly or for a prolonged period.

STOPPING THE DRUG
Take rectal glycerin only as needed. However, you may stop using it if you are feeling better before the scheduled end of therapy.

PROLONGED USE
Prolonged, excessive use of glycerin may be associated with an increased risk of side effects, including laxative dependence. Therefore, do not use glycerin for more than 3 to 5 days unless your doctor instructs you to do otherwise.

▼ PRECAUTIONS

Over 60: Adverse reactions may be more likely and more severe in older patients.

Driving and Hazardous Work: Do not drive or engage in hazardous work until you determine how the medicine affects you.

Alcohol: No special precautions are required.

Pregnancy: Adequate human studies have not been done. Before taking glycerin, tell your doctor if you are or are planning to become pregnant.

Breast Feeding: Glycerin suppositories may be used safely by nursing mothers.

Infants and Children: Not recommended for use by children under age 6.

Special Concerns: A single missed bowel movement does not constitute constipation; do not use glycerin under such circumstances. Prolonged constipation or persistent rectal pain and discomfort should be evaluated by your doctor. Remember that chronic use of glycerin or any laxative can lead to laxative dependence. You should be sure to consume adequate amounts of bulk in your diet; good sources include bran or other cereals, fresh fruit, and vegetables.

OVERDOSE
Symptoms: No specific ones have been reported.

What to Do: An overdose of glycerin is unlikely to be life-threatening. However, if someone takes a much larger dose than prescribed, call your doctor.

▼ INTERACTIONS

DRUG INTERACTIONS
No significant drug interactions have been reported.

FOOD INTERACTIONS
No known food interactions.

DISEASE INTERACTIONS
Caution is advised when taking glycerin laxatives. Consult your doctor if you have any of the following: abdominal pain and fever, rectal bleeding, ostomy (an artificial surgical opening in the body to allow the release of urine or feces), diabetes mellitus, heart or kidney disease, or high blood pressure.

☰ SIDE EFFECTS ☰
⬇ ⬇

SERIOUS
There are no serious side effects associated with the use of glycerin rectal.

COMMON
Cramping.

LESS COMMON
Rectal pain, itching, or burning sensation. This is thought to be more common with dosage forms that require an applicator. If you notice increased pain or bleeding from the rectum after use of glycerin products, call your doctor. Weakness, sweating, and symptoms of dehydration (thirst, dizziness) also may occur.

GUAIFENESIN

Available in: Capsules, tablets, oral solution, syrup, extended-release forms
Available as Generic? Yes
Drug Class: Expectorant

▼ USAGE INFORMATION

WHY IT'S TAKEN
Guaifenesin is classified as an expectorant; that is, it is designed to reduce the thickness of mucus and phlegm, making it easier to cough up and out of the lungs and so improve breathing. It is used to treat minor upper respiratory infections and related conditions, such as bronchitis, colds, and sinus or throat infections. Guaifenesin is not a cough suppressant, and despite its popularity and its FDA approval as an expectorant, there is little scientific evidence that it is truly effective at reducing the thickness of mucus.

HOW IT WORKS
Guaifenesin supposedly increases the production of fluids in the respiratory tract and helps to liquefy and thin mucus secretions.

▼ DOSAGE GUIDELINES

RANGE AND FREQUENCY
Adults—Capsules, tablets, oral solution, syrup: 200 to 400 mg every 4 hours, to a maximum of 2,400 mg a day. Extended-release capsules and tablets: 600 to 1,200 mg every 12 hours, to a maximum of 2,400 mg a day. Children 2 to 12 years of age—Consult your doctor.

ONSET OF EFFECT
Usually within several hours.

DURATION OF ACTION
The exact duration of action is not known.

DIETARY ADVICE
Maintain your usual food and fluid intake. Increase fluids if you have a fever or diarrhea. Coughing also increases your daily fluid requirements.

STORAGE
Store in a tightly sealed container away from heat and direct light. Keep liquid forms of guaifenesin refrigerated, but do not allow it to freeze. Keep away from moisture and extremes in temperature.

MISSED DOSE
Take it as soon as you remember. If it is near the time for the next dose, skip the missed dose and resume your regular dosage schedule. Do not double the next dose.

STOPPING THE DRUG
You may stop taking guaifenesin before the scheduled end of therapy if you are feeling better; otherwise, take as prescribed for the full treatment period.

PROLONGED USE
Therapy with guaifenesin is usually completed within 7 to 10 days. If you have a persistent cough, you may need special evaluation. Do not take nonprescription guaifenesin for more than 7 days without the approval of your doctor.

▼ PRECAUTIONS

Over 60: Adverse reactions may be more likely and more severe in this group.

Driving and Hazardous Work: Do not drive or engage in hazardous work until you determine how the medicine affects you.

Alcohol: No special warnings.

Pregnancy: Thorough studies have not been done, although no serious problems have been reported; consult your doctor for advice.

Breast Feeding: Guaifenesin may pass into breast milk, although no problems have been documented. Consult your doctor for advice.

Infants and Children: Generally, it should not be given to children under 2 unless directed otherwise by a pediatrician; children under 12 who have a persistent cough should be examined by a doctor before they are given guaifenesin.

Special Concerns: Guaifenesin is present in numerous nonprescription cough and cold remedies, so ask your pharmacist if you are unsure whether a product you are buying contains it. Do not treat a persistent cough on your own for more than a week or so without seeking medical advice. Avoid giving capsules or tablets to young children, since it is difficult to rely on children to swallow these dosage forms in one piece. Capsules and tablets should not be chewed.

OVERDOSE
Symptoms: No specific ones have been reported.

What to Do: An overdose of guaifenesin is unlikely to be life-threatening. However, if someone takes a much larger dose than prescribed, call your doctor, emergency medical services (EMS), or the nearest poison control center.

▼ INTERACTIONS

DRUG INTERACTIONS
None reported.

FOOD INTERACTIONS
None reported.

DISEASE INTERACTIONS
None reported.

≡ SIDE EFFECTS ≡

SERIOUS
No serious side effects are associated with guaifenesin.

COMMON
No common side effects are associated with guaifenesin.

LESS COMMON
Diarrhea; dizziness; headache; abdominal pain, nausea, or vomiting; skin rash; itching; hives.

HYDROCORTISONE TOPICAL

Available in: Cream, lotion, ointment, topical solution, dental paste
Available as Generic? Yes
Drug Class: Topical corticosteroid

BRAND NAMES

Acticort 100, Aeroseb-HC, Ala-Cort, Ala-Scalp HP, Allercort, Alphaderm, Anusol, Anusol-HC, Bactine, Beta HC, CaldeCORT Anti-Itch, Cetacort, Cort-Dome, Cortaid, Cortifair, Cortril, Delacort, Dermacort, DermiCort, Dermtex HC, Gly-Cort, Gynecort, Hi-Cor 2.5, Hydro-Tex, Hytone, LactiCare-HC, Lanacort, Lemoderm, Locoid, My Cort, Nutracort, Orabase-HCA, Pentacort, Rederm, S-T Cort, Synacort, Texacort, Westcort

▼ USAGE INFORMATION

WHY IT'S TAKEN
To treat certain skin conditions that are associated with itching, redness, scaling and peeling, pain, and other signs of inflammation. It is also used to treat inflammatory conditions within the mouth.

HOW IT WORKS
Topical hydrocortisone appears to interfere with the formation of natural substances within the body that are directly responsible for the process of inflammation, which produces swelling, redness, and pain.

▼ DOSAGE GUIDELINES

RANGE AND FREQUENCY
Adults using dental paste: Apply at bedtime to affected areas of the mouth. Adults using cream, lotion, ointment, solution: Apply sparingly to affected areas of the skin 1 to 2 (sometimes 3) times daily. Children: Consult your pediatrician for specific dosage and other advice.

ONSET OF EFFECT
Steroids begin to exert their effect soon after application. However, recognizable changes in your condition may take several days or more to develop.

DURATION OF ACTION
Unknown.

DIETARY ADVICE
Maintain your usual food and fluid intake.

STORAGE
Store in a tightly sealed container away from heat and direct light. Keep away from moisture and extremes in temperature.

MISSED DOSE
Apply it as soon as you remember. If it is near the time for the next dose, skip the missed dose and resume your regular dosage schedule. Do not double the next dose.

STOPPING THE DRUG
Take as prescribed for the full treatment period, even if you begin to feel better before the scheduled end of therapy.

PROLONGED USE
Therapy with this medication may require weeks or months; long-term therapy requires monitoring by your physician even with a low-potency product.

▼ PRECAUTIONS

Over 60: Adverse reactions to this medication may be more likely and more severe; therapy with topical corticosteroids should therefore be brief and infrequent.

Driving and Hazardous Work: The use of hydrocortisone topical preparation should not impair your ability to perform such tasks safely.

Alcohol: No special precautions are necessary.

Pregnancy: It should not be used for prolonged periods in pregnant women or in those trying to become pregnant.

Breast Feeding: Although problems have not been documented, caution is advised. Do not apply to breasts prior to nursing. Consult your doctor for specific advice.

Infants and Children: Not recommended for prolonged use. Consult your pediatrician.

Special Concerns: Avoid use of this medication around the eye. Hydrocortisone is not a treatment for acne, burns, infections, or disorders of pigmentation. Do not bandage or wrap the medicated area of skin with any special dressings or coverings unless specifically told to do so by your doctor.

OVERDOSE
Symptoms: No specific ones have been reported.

What to Do: An overdose is unlikely to be life-threatening. However, in the event of accidental ingestion or apparent overdose, call your doctor, emergency medical services (EMS), or the nearest poison control immediately.

▼ INTERACTIONS

DRUG INTERACTIONS
None reported.

FOOD INTERACTIONS
None reported.

DISEASE INTERACTIONS
Consult your doctor before taking this medication if you have any of the following medical conditions: diabetes; skin infection, or skin sores and ulcers; infection at another site in your body; tuberculosis; unusual bleeding or bruising; glaucoma; or cataracts.

≡ SIDE EFFECTS ≡

SERIOUS
Serious side effects from the use of topical hydrocortisone are very rare.

COMMON
Burning, itching, irritation, redness, dryness, acne, stinging and cracking of skin, numbness or tingling in the extremities (in 0.5% to 1% of patients).

LESS COMMON
Blistering and pus near hair follicles, unusual bleeding or easy bruising, darkening or prominence of small surface veins, increased susceptibility to infection.

IBUPROFEN

BRAND NAMES

Advil, Advil Liqui-Gels, Excedrin IB, Genpril, Haltran, Ibu-Tab, Ibuprin, Ibuprohm, Medipren, Midol IB, Motrin, Nuprin, Pamprin-IB, Rufen, Trendar

Available in: Tablets, oral solution, chewable tablets
Available as Generic? Yes
Drug Class: Nonsteroidal anti-inflammatory drug (NSAID)

▼ USAGE INFORMATION

WHY IT'S TAKEN
To treat mild to moderate pain and inflammation caused by tendinitis, arthritis, bursitis, gout, soft tissue injuries, migraine and other vascular headaches, menstrual cramps, and other conditions. It is also used to reduce fever.

HOW IT WORKS
NSAIDs work by interfering with the formation of prostaglandins, substances that cause inflammation and make nerves more sensitive to pain impulses. NSAIDs also have other modes of action that are less well understood.

▼ DOSAGE GUIDELINES

RANGE AND FREQUENCY
Adults—For mild to moderate pain, arthritis, and menstrual pain: 200 to 400 mg every 4 to 6 hours. For fever: 200 to 400 mg every 4 to 6 hours, but not more than 1,200 mg a day. Children ages 6 months to 12 years— For fevers below 102.5°F, 5 mg for every 2.2 lbs (1 kg) of body weight every 6 to 8 hours. For higher fevers, 10 mg per 2.2 lbs every 6 to 8 hours, but not more than 40 mg per 2.2 lbs a day.

ONSET OF EFFECT
For pain and fever, 30 minutes. For arthritis, up to 3 weeks.

DURATION OF ACTION
4 hours or more.

DIETARY ADVICE
Take ibuprofen with food.

STORAGE
Store in a tightly sealed container away from moisture, heat, and direct light.

MISSED DOSE
Take it as soon as you remember. However, if it is near the time for the next dose, skip the missed dose and resume your regular dosage schedule. Do not double the next dose.

STOPPING THE DRUG
If your doctor has told you to take this drug, do not stop without consulting him or her.

PROLONGED USE
Prolonged use can cause gastrointestinal problems, which may include ulceration and bleeding, kidney dysfunction, and liver inflammation. See your doctor regularly for laboratory tests and examinations.

▼ PRECAUTIONS

Over 60: Because of the potentially greater consequences of gastrointestinal side effects, the dose of NSAIDs for older patients, especially those over age 70, is often cut in half.

Driving and Hazardous Work: Do not drive or engage in hazardous work until you determine how the medicine affects you.

Alcohol: Avoid alcohol, as it may increase the risk of stomach irritation.

Pregnancy: Avoid or discontinue this drug if you are pregnant or are planning to become pregnant.

Breast Feeding: Ibuprofen passes into breast milk; avoid use while nursing.

Infants and Children: May be used in exceptional circumstances; consult your doctor.

Special Concerns: Because NSAIDs can interfere with blood coagulation, this drug should be stopped at least 3 days prior to any surgery.

OVERDOSE
Symptoms: Severe nausea, vomiting, headache, confusion, seizures.

What to Do: Call your doctor, emergency medical services (EMS), or the nearest poison control center immediately.

▼ INTERACTIONS

DRUG INTERACTIONS
Do not take this drug with aspirin or any other NSAIDs without your doctor's approval. In addition, consult your doctor if you are taking antihypertensives, steroids, anticoagulants, antibiotics, itraconazole or ketoconazole, plicamycin, penicillamine, valproic acid, phenytoin, cyclosporine, digitalis drugs, lithium, methotrexate, probenecid, triamterene, or zidovudine.

FOOD INTERACTIONS
No known food interactions.

DISEASE INTERACTIONS
Consult your doctor if you have any of the following: bleeding problems, gastrointestinal inflammation or ulcers, diabetes mellitus, systemic lupus erythematosus (SLE, lupus), anemia, asthma, epilepsy, Parkinson's disease, kidney stones, or a history of heart disease or alcohol abuse. Use of ibuprofen may cause complications in patients with liver or kidney disease, since these organs work together to remove the medication from the body.

≡ SIDE EFFECTS ≡

SERIOUS
Shortness of breath or wheezing, with or without swelling of legs or other signs of heart failure; chest pain; peptic ulcer disease with vomiting of blood; black, tarry stools; decreasing kidney function. Call your doctor immediately.

COMMON
Nausea, vomiting, heartburn, diarrhea, constipation, headache, dizziness, sleepiness.

LESS COMMON
Ulcers or sores in mouth, depression, rashes or blistering of skin, ringing sound in the ears, unusual tingling or numbness of the hands or feet, seizures, blurred vision. Also: elevated potassium levels, decreased blood counts; such problems can be detected by your doctor.

INSULIN (INTERMEDIATE-ACTING, NPH, LENTE)

BRAND NAMES

Humulin L, Humulin N, Insulatard NPH (purified pork), Insulated NPH Human, Lente Iletin I (beef and pork), Lente Iletin II (purified beef), Lente Iletin II (purified pork), Novolin L, Novolin L Pen-Fill Cartridges, Novolin N, NPH Iletin I (beef and pork), NPH Iletin II (purified beef), NPH Iletin II (purified pork)

Available in: Injection
Available as Generic? No
Drug Class: Antidiabetic agent

▼ USAGE INFORMATION

WHY IT'S TAKEN
For long-term treatment of diabetes mellitus. All patients with type 1 diabetes require lifelong insulin treatment. Patients with type 2 diabetes may require insulin if they are unable to control their blood glucose (sugar) levels with diet and oral medications.

HOW IT WORKS
Insulin, a hormone secreted by the beta cells of the pancreas, plays an essential role in controlling the metabolism and storage of carbohydrates, fat, and protein. Insulin is secreted in response to a rise in blood sugar (glucose). Insulin lowers blood glucose by increasing its uptake by body cells, especially muscle, and by reducing the release of glucose from the liver between meals.

▼ DOSAGE GUIDELINES

RANGE AND FREQUENCY
Injected 1 or 2 times a day. Doses and frequency are determined by your doctor. Intermediate-acting (NPH or Lente) insulin can be mixed in the same syringe with rapid-acting insulin; draw up the rapid-acting insulin first. Intermediate-acting insulin solutions are cloudy (insulin settles to the bottom of the bottle) and must be rolled or gently shaken to distribute the insulin evenly in the solution before drawing it up into the syringe.

ONSET OF EFFECT
Within 1 hour; peak effect occurs within 8 to 12 hours.

DURATION OF ACTION
From 12 to 18 hours.

DIETARY ADVICE
All patients with diabetes should follow the general dietary recommendations of the American Diabetes Association. Though intake of simple sugars is not forbidden, consuming a large amount of sugary foods at one time may trigger a rapid rise in blood glucose that can increase urination and thirst. In addition, patients who take insulin must remain consistent from day to day in the timing and caloric content of their meals. Depending on the timing, dose, and types of insulin prescribed, snacks may be recommended in the late afternoon, before bedtime, or prior to unusual physical activity. Patients with diabetes must always have available a juice, food, or tablets that can raise their blood glucose levels rapidly to counter an episode of hypoglycemia.

STORAGE
Refrigerate insulin but do not allow it to freeze. Insulin does not have to be kept refrigerated when you're traveling for short periods, but exposure to high temperatures must be avoided.

MISSED DOSE
Timing of insulin doses is extremely important. The best approach is to measure blood glucose and add a dose of regular insulin if your glucose levels are too high. Otherwise, wait for the next dose on your schedule.

STOPPING THE DRUG
Do not stop taking insulin injections unless ordered by your doctor. Patients with diabetes are often given general instructions for modifying their insulin doses based on repeated home blood glucose measurements.

PROLONGED USE
After many years with diabetes, some patients become insensitive to the symptoms of hypoglycemia and are at risk for serious brain complications caused by prolonged, unrecognized hypoglycemia.

▼ PRECAUTIONS

Over 60: No special warnings. Some older people may, however, have vision problems that may make it difficult to draw up the correct dose of insulin.

Driving and Hazardous Work: Patients taking insulin must be very careful to avoid hypoglycemia when driving or engaging in hazardous work.

Alcohol: Moderate alcohol intake, especially when taken with large meals, does not adversely affect control of diabetes or alter the dose of insulin. However, large amounts of alcohol increase the risk of hypoglycemia.

Pregnancy: Strict metabolic control—using insulin injections in most women—must

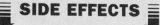

☰ SIDE EFFECTS ☰

SERIOUS
Symptoms of hypoglycemia can be caused by the release of adrenaline or by an inadequate supply of glucose to the brain. With severe hypoglycemia, lack of sufficient glucose to the brain may cause slurred speech, impaired concentration, confusion, seizures, coma, irreversible brain damage, and death. Mild hypoglycemia may cause restless sleep, nightmares, or a cold sweat that awakens patients at night.

COMMON
Symptoms resulting from the release of adrenaline are common with mild to moderate hypoglycemia. They include cold sweats, anxiety, shakiness, hunger, rapid heartbeat, and headache. Weight gain is also common when taking insulin.

LESS COMMON
Allergic reactions, lipoatrophy (depressions in the skin due to loss of fat tissue), and lipohypertrophy (excessive accumulation of fat tissue).

be maintained during pregnancy to reduce the risk of birth defects, fetal complications, or death at the time of delivery. In women who had diabetes before the onset of pregnancy, the dose of insulin is often smaller during the first third (trimester) of pregnancy and then higher during the final two trimesters. When women first develop diabetes during pregnancy (gestational diabetes), insulin requirements drop rapidly after delivery and most do not need to continue with insulin treatment.

Breast Feeding: Insulin requirements tend to be lower during breast feeding. Home glucose monitoring is important to avoid hypoglycemia. Insulin is not present in breast milk.

Infants and Children: Treatment with insulin in children is the same as in older people with diabetes.

Special Concerns: Inadequate amounts of insulin in type 1 diabetes may lead to the serious complication of diabetic ketoacidosis, characterized by loss of appetite, excessive thirst and urination, nausea, vomiting, deep breathing, fruity breath odor, drowsiness, confusion, and loss of consciousness.

OVERDOSE

Symptoms: Insulin overdose results in hypoglycemia (see Side Effects for symptoms).

What to Do: For mild to moderate hypoglycemia, ingest drinks or food containing sugar. For more severe hypoglycemia, administer injections of glucagon or call emergency medical services (EMS) immediately.

▼ **INTERACTIONS**

DRUG INTERACTIONS
A large number of drugs can promote either elevated blood glucose levels or hypoglycemia. Be sure that your doctor knows about all of the medications you take and is informed before you start taking any new drugs, either by prescription or over the counter. Corticosteroids in particular are likely to raise blood glucose levels and insulin requirements. Beta-blockers (commonly used for hypertension) may cause either high blood glucose levels or hypoglycemia; in addition, because these medications may dampen the symptoms of hypoglycemia that are caused by adrenaline release, mild degrees of hypoglycemia may progress unnoticed to more serious hypoglycemia affecting the brain.

FOOD INTERACTIONS
Insulin requirements are increased when larger amounts of calories are ingested, especially simple sugars and carbohydrates.

DISEASE INTERACTIONS
Insulin requirements are increased by infections, psychological stress, or an uncontrolled overactive thyroid, and often at a time of surgery. Requirements may diminish with kidney disease or an underactive adrenal or pituitary gland.

INSULIN (LONG-ACTING, ULTRALENTE)

Available in: Injection
Available as Generic? No
Drug Class: Antidiabetic agent

▼ USAGE INFORMATION

WHY IT'S TAKEN
For long-term treatment of diabetes mellitus. All patients with type 1 diabetes require lifelong insulin treatment. Patients with type 2 diabetes may require insulin if they are unable to control their blood glucose (sugar) levels with diet and oral medications.

HOW IT WORKS
Insulin, a hormone secreted by the beta cells of the pancreas, plays an essential role in controlling the metabolism and storage of carbohydrates, fat, and protein. Insulin is secreted in response to a rise in blood sugar (glucose). Insulin lowers blood glucose by increasing its uptake by body cells, especially muscle, and by reducing the release of glucose from the liver between meals.

▼ DOSAGE GUIDELINES

RANGE AND FREQUENCY
Injected 1 or 2 times a day. Doses and frequency are determined by your doctor. Long-acting (Ultralente) insulin can be mixed in the same syringe with rapid-acting insulin. Start by drawing up the rapid-acting insulin first. Long-acting insulin solutions are cloudy (insulin settles to the bottom of the bottle) and must be rolled or gently shaken to distribute the insulin evenly in the solution before drawing it up into the syringe.

ONSET OF EFFECT
It begins to take effect within 6 to 8 hours; the peak effect occurs within 10 to 20 hours of injection.

DURATION OF ACTION
From 24 to 36 hours.

DIETARY ADVICE
All patients with diabetes should follow the general dietary recommendations of the American Diabetes Association. Though intake of simple sugars is not forbidden, consuming a large amount of sugary foods at one time may trigger a rapid rise in blood glucose that can increase urination and thirst. In addition, patients who take insulin must remain consistent from day to day in the timing and caloric content of their meals. Depending on the timing, dose, and types of insulin prescribed, snacks may be recommended in the late afternoon, before bedtime, or prior to unusual physical activity. Patients with diabetes must always have available a juice, food, or tablets that can raise their blood glucose levels rapidly to counter an episode of hypoglycemia.

STORAGE
Refrigerate insulin but do not allow it to freeze. Insulin does not have to be kept refrigerated when you're traveling for short periods, but exposure to high temperatures makes it unusable.

MISSED DOSE
Timing of insulin doses is extremely important. The best approach is to measure blood glucose and add a dose of regular insulin if your glucose levels are too high. Otherwise, wait for the next dose on your schedule.

STOPPING THE DRUG
Do not stop taking insulin injections unless ordered by your doctor. Patients with diabetes are often given general instructions for modifying

their insulin doses based on repeated home blood glucose measurements.

PROLONGED USE
After many years with diabetes, some patients become insensitive to the symptoms of hypoglycemia and are at risk for serious brain complications due to prolonged, unrecognized hypoglycemia.

▼ PRECAUTIONS

Over 60: No special warnings. Some older people may, however, have vision problems that may make it difficult to draw up the correct dose of insulin.

Driving and Hazardous Work: Patients taking insulin must be very careful to avoid hypoglycemia when driving or engaging in hazardous work.

Alcohol: Moderate alcohol intake, especially when taken with large meals, does not adversely affect control of diabetes or alter the dose of insulin. However, large amounts of alcohol increase the risk of hypoglycemia.

Pregnancy: Strict metabolic control—using insulin injections in most women—must be maintained during pregnancy to reduce the risk of birth defects, fetal complications, or death at the time of delivery. In women who had diabetes before the onset of pregnancy, the dose of insulin is often smaller during the first third (trimester) of pregnancy and then higher during the final two trimesters. When women first develop

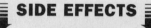

SIDE EFFECTS

SERIOUS
Symptoms of hypoglycemia can be caused by the release of adrenaline or by an inadequate supply of glucose to the brain. With severe hypoglycemia, lack of sufficient glucose to the brain may cause slurred speech, impaired concentration, confusion, seizures, coma, irreversible brain damage, and death. Mild hypoglycemia may cause restless sleep, nightmares, or a cold sweat that awakens patients at night.

COMMON
Symptoms resulting from release of adrenaline are common manifestations of mild to moderate hypoglycemia. They include cold sweats, anxiety, shakiness, hunger, rapid heartbeat, headache, and nervousness. Weight gain is common when taking insulin.

LESS COMMON
Allergic reactions, lipoatrophy (depressions in the skin due to loss of fat tissue), and lipohypertrophy (excessive accumulation of fat tissue).

diabetes during pregnancy (gestational diabetes), insulin requirements drop rapidly after delivery and most do not need to continue with insulin treatment.

Breast Feeding: Insulin requirements tend to be lower during breast feeding. Home glucose monitoring is important to avoid hypoglycemia. Breast milk does not contain insulin.

Infants and Children: Treatment with insulin in young patients is the same as that in older people with diabetes.

Special Concerns: Inadequate amounts of insulin in type 1

diabetes may lead to the serious complication of diabetic ketoacidosis, characterized by loss of appetite, excessive thirst and urination, nausea, vomiting, deep breathing, fruity breath odor, drowsiness, confusion, and loss of consciousness.

OVERDOSE

Symptoms: Insulin overdose results in hypoglycemia (see Side Effects for symptoms).

What to Do: For mild to moderate hypoglycemia, ingest drinks or food containing sugar. For more severe hypoglycemia, administer injections of glucagon or call emergency medical services (EMS) immediately.

▼ INTERACTIONS

DRUG INTERACTIONS
A large number of drugs can promote either elevated blood glucose levels or hypoglycemia. Be sure that your doctor knows about all of the medications you take and is informed before you start taking any new drugs, either by prescription or over the counter. Corticosteroids in particular are likely to raise blood glucose levels and insulin requirements. Beta-blockers (commonly used for hypertension) may cause either high blood glucose levels or hypoglycemia; in addition, because these drugs may dampen the symptoms of hypoglycemia that are

caused by adrenaline release, mild degrees of hypoglycemia may progress unnoticed to more serious hypoglycemia affecting the brain.

FOOD INTERACTIONS
Insulin requirements are increased when larger amounts of calories are ingested, especially simple sugars and carbohydrates.

DISEASE INTERACTIONS
Insulin requirements are increased by infections, psychological stress, or an uncontrolled overactive thyroid, and often at a time of surgery. Requirements may diminish with kidney disease or an underactive adrenal or pituitary gland.

INSULIN (REGULAR, RAPID-ACTING, OR SEMILENTE)

Available in: Injection
Available as Generic? No
Drug Class: Antidiabetic agent

BRAND NAMES

Humulin BR, Humulin R, Novolin R, Novolin R Pen-Fill Cartridges, Regular Iletin I (beef and pork), Regular Iletin II (purified beef), Regular Iletin II (purified pork), Semilente Iletin I (beef and pork), Semilente Insulin (beef), Velosulin Human, Velosulin (purified pork)

▼ USAGE INFORMATION

WHY IT'S TAKEN
For long-term treatment of diabetes mellitus. All patients with type 1 diabetes require lifelong insulin treatment. Patients with type 2 diabetes may require insulin if they are unable to control their blood glucose (sugar) levels with diet and oral medications.

HOW IT WORKS
Insulin, a hormone secreted by the beta cells of the pancreas, plays an essential role in controlling the metabolism and storage of carbohydrates, fat, and protein. Insulin is secreted in response to a rise in blood sugar (glucose). Insulin lowers blood glucose by increasing its uptake by body cells, especially muscle, and by reducing the release of glucose from the liver between meals.

▼ DOSAGE GUIDELINES

RANGE AND FREQUENCY
It may be taken 1 to 4 times daily, before meals and possibly at bedtime. Doses and frequency are determined by your doctor. Regular (or rapid-acting or semilente) insulin should be administered 30 to 45 minutes before a meal. It can be mixed in the same syringe with intermediate-acting insulins. Draw up the regular insulin first.

ONSET OF EFFECT
It begins to take effect within 45 minutes; peak effect occurs within 2 to 4 hours.

DURATION OF ACTION
From 4 to 6 hours.

DIETARY ADVICE
All patients with diabetes should follow the general dietary recommendations of the American Diabetes Association. Though intake of simple sugars is not forbidden, consuming a large amount of sugary foods at one time may trigger a rapid rise in blood glucose that can increase urination and thirst. In addition, patients who take insulin must remain consistent from day to day in the timing and caloric content of their meals. Depending on the timing, dose, and types of insulin prescribed, snacks may be recommended in the late afternoon, before bedtime, or prior to unusual physical activity. Patients with diabetes must always have available a juice, food, or tablets that can raise their blood glucose levels rapidly to counter an episode of hypoglycemia.

STORAGE
Refrigerate insulin but do not allow it to freeze. Insulin does not have to be kept refrigerated when you're traveling for short periods, but exposure to high temperatures must always be avoided.

MISSED DOSE
Timing of insulin doses is extremely important. The best approach is to measure blood glucose and add a dose of regular insulin if glucose levels are too high. Otherwise, wait for the next scheduled dose.

STOPPING THE DRUG
Do not stop taking insulin injections unless ordered by your doctor. Patients with diabetes are often given general instructions for modifying their insulin doses based on home blood glucose measurements.

PROLONGED USE
After many years with diabetes, some patients become insensitive to the symptoms of hypoglycemia and are at risk for serious brain complications due to prolonged, unrecognized hypoglycemia.

▼ PRECAUTIONS

Over 60: No special warnings. Some older people may, however, have vision problems that may make it difficult to draw up the correct dose of insulin.

Driving and Hazardous Work: Patients taking insulin must be very careful to avoid hypoglycemia when driving or engaging in hazardous work.

Alcohol: Moderate alcohol intake, especially when taken with large meals, does not adversely affect control of diabetes or alter the dose of insulin. However, large amounts of alcohol increase the risk of hypoglycemia.

Pregnancy: Strict metabolic control—using insulin injections in most women—must be maintained during pregnancy to reduce the risk of birth defects, fetal complications, or death at the time of delivery. In women who had diabetes before the onset of

≣ SIDE EFFECTS ≣

⬇ SERIOUS ⬇
Symptoms of hypoglycemia can be caused by the release of adrenaline or by an inadequate supply of glucose to the brain. With severe hypoglycemia, lack of sufficient glucose to the brain may cause slurred speech, impaired concentration, confusion, seizures, coma, irreversible brain damage, and death. Mild hypoglycemia may cause restless sleep, nightmares, or a cold sweat that awakens patients at night.

COMMON
Symptoms resulting from release of adrenaline are common manifestations of mild to moderate hypoglycemia. They include cold sweats, anxiety, shakiness, hunger, rapid heartbeat, headache, and nervousness. Weight gain is common when taking insulin.

LESS COMMON
Allergic reactions, lipoatrophy (depressions in the skin due to loss of fat tissue), and lipohypertrophy (excessive accumulation of fat tissue).

pregnancy, the dose of insulin is often smaller during the first third (trimester) of pregnancy and then higher during the final two trimesters. When women first develop diabetes during pregnancy (gestational diabetes), insulin requirements drop rapidly after delivery and most do not need to continue with insulin treatment.

Breast Feeding: Insulin requirements tend to be lower during breast feeding. Home glucose monitoring is important to avoid hypoglycemia. Breast milk does not contain insulin.

Infants and Children: Treatment with insulin in young patients is the same as that in older people with diabetes.

Special Concerns: Inadequate amounts of insulin in type 1 diabetes may lead to the serious complication of diabetic ketoacidosis, characterized by loss of appetite, excessive thirst and urination, nausea, vomiting, deep breathing, fruity breath odor, drowsiness, confusion, and loss of consciousness.

OVERDOSE

Symptoms: Insulin overdose results in hypoglycemia (see Side Effects for symptoms).

What to Do: For mild to moderate hypoglycemia, ingest drinks or food containing sugar. For more severe hypoglycemia, administer injections of glucagon or call emergency medical services (EMS) immediately.

▼ INTERACTIONS

DRUG INTERACTIONS

A large number of drugs can promote either elevated blood glucose levels or hypoglycemia. Be sure that your doctor knows about all of the medications you take and is informed before you start taking any new drugs, either over the counter or by prescription. Corticosteroids in particular are likely to raise blood glucose levels and insulin requirements. Beta-blockers (commonly used to treat hypertension) may cause either high blood glucose levels or hypoglycemia; in addition, because these medications may dampen the symptoms of hypoglycemia that are caused by adrenaline release, mild degrees of hypoglycemia may progress unnoticed to more serious hypoglycemia affecting the brain.

FOOD INTERACTIONS

Insulin requirements are increased when larger amounts of calories are ingested, especially simple sugars and carbohydrates.

DISEASE INTERACTIONS

Insulin requirements are increased by infections, psychological stress, or an uncontrolled overactive thyroid, and often at a time of surgery. Requirements may diminish with kidney disease or an underactive adrenal or pituitary gland.

IODINE TOPICAL

Iodine Tincture, Iodopen

Available in: Topical solution
Available as Generic? Yes
Drug Class: Antibacterial (topical); antiseptic

▼ USAGE INFORMATION

WHY IT'S TAKEN
Iodine is a very effective disinfectant used for prevention and treatment of minor skin infections caused by bacteria. It is also used to disinfect the skin prior to needle procedures and minor surgeries (such as blood drawing, dialysis, and injections).

HOW IT WORKS
Iodine poisons bacteria on contact, by causing the proteins comprising the organism to congeal.

▼ DOSAGE GUIDELINES

RANGE AND FREQUENCY
Adults: Apply to affected site as directed by a physician or according to manufacturer's instructions on the label. Children 1 month of age and over: Consult a pediatrician.

ONSET OF EFFECT
Immediate.

DURATION OF ACTION
Unknown.

DIETARY ADVICE
Maintain your usual food and fluid intake. Increase fluids if you have a fever or diarrhea, in hot weather, or during exercise.

STORAGE
Store in a tightly sealed container away from heat and direct light. Keep iodine away from moisture and extremes in temperature.

MISSED DOSE
Apply as soon as you remember. If it is near the time for the next dose, skip the missed dose and resume your regular dosage schedule.

STOPPING THE DRUG
Use as prescribed for the full treatment period, even if you begin to feel better before the scheduled end of therapy.

PROLONGED USE
Therapy with this medication should be concluded within 7 to 10 days. Consult your physician if your condition has not improved—and especially if it has worsened—at any time after starting therapy with iodine.

▼ PRECAUTIONS

Over 60: No special problems are expected.

Driving and Hazardous Work: The use of iodine should not impair your ability to perform such tasks safely.

Alcohol: No special precautions are necessary.

Pregnancy: Avoid or discontinue using iodine if you are pregnant or trying to become pregnant.

Breast Feeding: Iodine passes into breast milk; avoid or discontinue usage while nursing.

Infants and Children: Iodine is not recommended for use on children younger than 1 month of age.

Special Concerns: Iodine has serious side effects if it is absorbed in large amounts into your blood. Therefore, do not apply excessive amounts to affected skin. Do not swallow iodine solutions. Above all, never apply this medication to open wounds, to deep cuts, or to bleeding or ulcerated skin. Do not use this medication near your eyes and be careful when applying iodine to the skin of your forehead or cheeks. Use small quantities and apply them carefully, instead of pouring on a large volume. If iodine gets into your eyes, wash with water immediately.

OVERDOSE
Symptoms: Overdose with topical iodine is unlikely when used as directed. Swallowing this medication may cause such symptoms as diarrhea, abdominal pain, nausea, vomiting, fever, excessive thirst, and decreased passage of urine.

What to Do: Call your doctor, emergency medical services (EMS), or the nearest poison control center immediately.

▼ INTERACTIONS

DRUG INTERACTIONS
No specific drug interactions have yet been documented. If you are concerned about whether a prescription or nonprescription medication you are taking may interact with topical iodine, consult your doctor or pharmacist for current information.

FOOD INTERACTIONS
No known food interactions.

DISEASE INTERACTIONS
Consult your doctor if you have any of the following: animal bites; large sores, blisters, ulcerations, or broken skin at the application site; severe injury at the application site; puncture wounds or other deep wounds; serious burns; or allergies to shellfish.

≡ SIDE EFFECTS ≡

SERIOUS
Used as directed, topical iodine is not expected to produce any serious side effects.

COMMON
Momentary burning or tingling at the site of application.

LESS COMMON
Irritation or skin allergy, with blistering, crusting, itching, or reddening of skin at site of application.

IPECAC SYRUP

Available in: Syrup
Available as Generic? Yes
Drug Class: Emetic

▼ USAGE INFORMATION

WHY IT'S TAKEN
To cause vomiting in persons who have ingested certain toxic substances or have taken an overdose of a drug.

HOW IT WORKS
Ipecac induces vomiting because it chemically irritates the stomach lining, which then triggers the body's vomiting reflex.

▼ DOSAGE GUIDELINES

RANGE AND FREQUENCY
Adults and teenagers: 15 to 30 ml, followed by 1 full glass of water. Children ages 1 to 12: 15 ml followed by ½ to 1 full glass of water. Children ages 6 months to 1 year: 5 to 10 ml, followed by ½ to 1 full glass of water. If vomiting does not occur, the first dose may be repeated one time after 20 minutes.

ONSET OF EFFECT
Within 20 to 30 minutes.

DURATION OF ACTION
From 20 to 25 minutes.

DIETARY ADVICE
Drink water immediately after taking ipecac syrup.

STORAGE
Store in a tightly sealed container away from moisture, heat, and direct light.

MISSED DOSE
Not applicable. It should be used more than 1 time only if clearly necessary.

STOPPING THE DRUG
Do not give more than 2 doses. If not effective, consult your doctor, emergency medical services (EMS), or local poison control center.

PROLONGED USE
Ipecac is not intended for prolonged use.

▼ PRECAUTIONS

Over 60: No special problems are expected.

Driving and Hazardous Work: Do not drive or engage in hazardous work until you determine how the drug affects you.

Alcohol: Avoid alcohol.

Pregnancy: No studies of the use of ipecac syrup during pregnancy have been done. Discuss with your doctor the relative risks and benefits of using it while pregnant.

Breast Feeding: Ipecac syrup may pass into breast milk; caution is advised. Consult your doctor for advice.

Infants and Children: Use by children should be under strict supervision. There is an increased risk of swallowing the vomited substance in children under 1 year of age. Consult your doctor before using ipecac syrup.

Special Concerns: Before giving ipecac syrup, consult your doctor, emergency medical services (EMS), or the nearest poison control center. Ipecac syrup should not be given to anyone who has ingested gasoline, paint thinner, kerosene, or a caustic substance such as lye. Do not give ipecac syrup to anyone who is unconscious or very drowsy, because of an increased risk that the vomited substance can enter the lung. If you have a child over 1 year of age in the house, keep 30 ml (1 oz) of ipecac syrup on hand for emergencies. Ipecac syrup should not be used to induce vomiting as a means of losing weight. It can be toxic to the heart.

OVERDOSE

Symptoms: Breathing difficulty, muscle stiffness, diarrhea.

What to Do: Call your doctor, emergency medical services (EMS), or the nearest poison control center immediately.

▼ INTERACTIONS

DRUG INTERACTIONS
Do not give any other medicines, including OTC drugs, with ipecac unless you first consult your doctor. Antiemetics can decrease the syrup's effect and increase its toxicity. If using activated charcoal, wait until the vomiting (induced by ipecac) has stopped before administering it.

FOOD INTERACTIONS
Ipecac syrup should not be taken with milk, milk products, or carbonated drinks. Milk and milk products prevent ipecac syrup from working properly. Carbonated beverages can cause the stomach to swell.

DISEASE INTERACTIONS
You should not take ipecac syrup if you suffer from or have heart disease, a history of seizures, shock, reduced gag reflex, drowsiness, or unconsciousness.

☰ SIDE EFFECTS ☰

SERIOUS
Heartbeat irregularities; nausea or vomiting lasting for more than 30 minutes; excessive diarrhea; weakness or stiffness of the muscles in the neck, arms, and legs; stomach pain or cramps; unusual fatigue; difficulty breathing. Call your doctor right away.

COMMON
Drowsiness and mild diarrhea.

LESS COMMON
There are no less-common side effects associated with the use of ipecac syrup.

KAOLIN WITH PECTIN

Available in: Oral suspension
Available as Generic? Yes
Drug Class: Antidiarrheal

▼ USAGE INFORMATION

WHY IT'S TAKEN
To treat diarrhea.

HOW IT WORKS
Kaolin with pectin absorbs fluids and binds to and removes bacteria and toxins from the digestive tract.

▼ DOSAGE GUIDELINES

RANGE AND FREQUENCY
Adults: 4 to 8 tablespoons (60 to 120 ml) after each loose bowel movement. Children age 12 and older: 3 to 4 tbsp (45 to 60 ml) after each loose bowel movement. Children ages 6 to 12: 2 to 4 tbsp (30 to 60 ml) after each loose bowel movement. Children ages 3 to 6: 1 to 2 tbsp (15 to 30 ml) after each loose bowel movement.

ONSET OF EFFECT
Unknown.

DURATION OF ACTION
Unknown.

DIETARY ADVICE
A mild diet is recommended when recovering from diarrhea. Bananas, rice, applesauce, and plain toast are good choices. Be sure to get plenty of fluids.

STORAGE
Store in a tightly sealed container away from moisture, heat, and direct light.

MISSED DOSE
Take it as soon as you remember. If it is nearly time for another dose, skip the missed dose. Do not double the next dose.

STOPPING THE DRUG
Do not use this drug for more than 2 days without consulting your doctor.

PROLONGED USE
This drug is not intended for prolonged use. Consult your doctor if diarrhea continues for more than 2 days.

▼ PRECAUTIONS

Over 60: Adverse reactions associated with diarrhea may be more severe in older patients. They should be sure to consume enough liquids to replace body fluids lost because of diarrhea.

Driving and Hazardous Work: The use of kaolin with pectin should not impair your ability to perform such tasks safely.

Alcohol: Avoid alcohol.

Pregnancy: It is not absorbed into the body and is not expected to cause problems during pregnancy.

Breast Feeding: It is not absorbed into the body and is not expected to cause problems during breast feeding.

Infants and Children: Kaolin with pectin should be used in children under the age of 3 only under the supervision of a doctor.

Special Concerns: In addition to taking medicine for diarrhea, it is important to replace the fluid lost by your body and to eat a proper diet. During the first 24 hours, drink plenty of caffeine-free clear liquids like water, broth, ginger ale, and decaffeinated tea. During the second 24 hours you may eat bland foods such as applesauce, bread, crackers, and oatmeal. Avoid caffeine, fried or spicy foods, bran, candy, fruits, and vegetables. They can make your condition worse.

OVERDOSE
Symptoms: Constipation.

What to Do: An overdose of kaolin with pectin is unlikely to be life-threatening. However, if someone takes a much larger dose than prescribed, call your doctor, emergency medical services (EMS), or the nearest poison control center immediately.

▼ INTERACTIONS

DRUG INTERACTIONS
Consult your doctor for specific advice if you are taking anticholinergics, antidyskinetics, digitalis drugs, lincomycins, loxapine, phenothiazines, thioxanthenes, or any other oral medication. Do not take any medication within 2 to 3 hours of taking kaolin with pectin.

FOOD INTERACTIONS
Fruits, fried or spicy foods, bran, candy, and caffeine-containing beverages can make diarrhea worse.

DISEASE INTERACTIONS
Caution is advised when taking kaolin with pectin. Consult your doctor if the diarrhea is suspected to be caused by parasites or dysentery.

≡ SIDE EFFECTS ≡

SERIOUS
No serious side effects have been reported.

COMMON
No common side effects have been reported.

LESS COMMON
Constipation.

KETOCONAZOLE TOPICAL

Available in: Cream, shampoo
Available as Generic? Yes
Drug Class: Topical antifungal

▼ USAGE INFORMATION

WHY IT'S TAKEN
Ketoconazole is used to treat fungal infections of the skin. These infections include tinea pedis (athlete's foot), tinea corporis (ringworm), tinea cruris (jock itch), yeast infections of the skin, seborrheic dermatitis, and others.

HOW IT WORKS
Ketoconazole prevents fungal organisms from manufacturing vital substances required for growth and function.

▼ DOSAGE GUIDELINES

RANGE AND FREQUENCY
Adults, for tinea and yeast: Apply once daily to affected skin. Treatment generally requires 2 to 6 weeks. Adults, for seborrheic dermatitis: Apply two times a day to affected skin. Treatment generally requires 4 weeks. Children: Consult your pediatrician.

ONSET OF EFFECT
Ketoconazole begins killing susceptible fungi shortly after contact. The effects may not be noticeable for several days or weeks.

DURATION OF ACTION
Unknown.

DIETARY ADVICE
Maintain your usual food and fluid intake. Increase fluid intake in hot weather, during exercise, or if you have a fever or diarrhea.

STORAGE
Store in a tightly sealed container away from heat and direct light.

MISSED DOSE
Apply it as soon as you remember. If it is near the time for the next dose, skip the missed dose and resume your regular dosage schedule. Do not double the next dose or apply an excessively thick film of topical medication to compensate for a missed application.

STOPPING THE DRUG
Apply ketoconazole as recommended for the full treatment period, even if you notice marked improvement before the scheduled end of the therapy.

PROLONGED USE
Therapy with this medication should not exceed 4 weeks.

▼ PRECAUTIONS

Over 60: Adverse reactions may be more likely and more severe in older patients.

Driving and Hazardous Work: The use of ketoconazole cream should not impair your ability to perform such tasks safely.

Alcohol: No special precautions are necessary.

Pregnancy: Avoid or discontinue use of ketoconazole if you are pregnant or trying to become pregnant.

Breast Feeding: Ketoconazole may pass into breast milk; avoid or discontinue usage while nursing. Consult your doctor for specific advice.

Infants and Children: Not recommended for use by young children.

Special Concerns: Avoid contact with eyes. Wash hands thoroughly after application. Tell your doctor if your condition has not improved within a few days of starting ketoconazole. As with any other antifungal, ketoconazole is useful only against organisms that are vulnerable to its effects. Therefore, it is important to tell your doctor if your condition has not improved—or has worsened—within a few days of starting ketoconazole. The particular organism causing your illness may be resistant to this medication.

▼ OVERDOSE

Symptoms: No specific ones have been reported.

What to Do: An overdose of ketoconazole is unlikely to be life-threatening. However, if someone applies a much larger dose than prescribed or ingests the medication, call your doctor, emergency medical services (EMS), or the nearest poison control center.

▼ INTERACTIONS

DRUG INTERACTIONS
No specific drug interactions are known as of this writing. If you are concerned about whether a prescription or over-the-counter medication you are taking may interact with ketoconazole, consult your physician or pharmacist for current information.

FOOD INTERACTIONS
No known food interactions.

DISEASE INTERACTIONS
Consult your physician if you have had previous allergies or an undesirable reaction to any other topical medication.

≣ SIDE EFFECTS ≣

SERIOUS
Blistering or ulceration of the skin; blistering of the lips, nose, and mouth.

COMMON
Brief burning, itching, or irritation after application of cream; peeling.

LESS COMMON
Severe burning, itching, swelling, increased redness, or any discomfort at the application site not present prior to therapy (as a result of allergic reaction).

KETOPROFEN

BRAND NAMES
Apo-Keto, Orudis, Oruvail, Rhodis

Available in: Tablets and capsules (also extended-release forms), rectal suppositories
Available as Generic? Yes
Drug Class: Nonsteroidal anti-inflammatory drug (NSAID)

▼ USAGE INFORMATION

WHY IT'S TAKEN
To treat mild to moderate pain and inflammation caused by tendinitis, arthritis, bursitis, gout, soft tissue injuries, migraine and other vascular headaches, menstrual cramps, and other conditions. When patients fail to respond to one NSAID, another may be tried. The greatest effectiveness often requires trial and error of several different NSAIDs.

HOW IT WORKS
NSAIDs work by interfering with the formation of prostaglandins, naturally occurring substances in the body that cause inflammation and make nerves more sensitive to pain impulses. NSAIDs also have other modes of action that are less well understood.

▼ DOSAGE GUIDELINES

RANGE AND FREQUENCY
Adults—Tablets or capsules: 50 mg, 4 times a day, or 75 mg, 3 times a day. Extended-release tablets or capsules: 200 mg once a day. Suppositories: 50 to 100 mg inserted twice a day (morning and evening). Sometimes, suppositories may be used only at night by people who take an oral dose during the day. Maximum dosage for all forms is 300 mg per day.

ONSET OF EFFECT
1 to 2 hours.

DURATION OF ACTION
3 to 4 hours.

DIETARY ADVICE
Take oral forms with food.

STORAGE
Store in a tightly sealed container away from moisture, heat, and direct light.

MISSED DOSE
Take it as soon as you remember. If it is near the time for the next dose, skip the missed dose and resume your regular dosage schedule. Do not double the next dose.

STOPPING THE DRUG
If your doctor has advised you to take this drug, do not stop without consulting him or her.

PROLONGED USE
Prolonged use can cause gastrointestinal ulceration and bleeding, kidney dysfunction, and liver inflammation. Consult your doctor about the need for medical examinations and laboratory studies.

▼ PRECAUTIONS

Over 60: Because of the potentially greater consequences of gastrointestinal side effects, the dose of NSAIDs for older patients, especially those over age 70, is often cut in half.

Driving and Hazardous Work: Do not drive or engage in hazardous work until you determine how the medicine affects you.

Alcohol: Avoid alcohol when using this medication because it increases the risk of stomach irritation.

Pregnancy: Do not use ketoprofen while pregnant.

Breast Feeding: Ketoprofen passes into breast milk; avoid use while nursing.

Infants and Children: Ketoprofen may be used in exceptional circumstances; consult your doctor.

Special Concerns: Because NSAIDs can interfere with blood coagulation, this drug should be stopped at least 3 days prior to any surgery.

OVERDOSE
Symptoms: Severe nausea, vomiting, headache, confusion, seizures.

What to Do: Call your doctor, emergency medical services (EMS), or the nearest poison control center immediately.

▼ INTERACTIONS

DRUG INTERACTIONS
Do not take this drug with aspirin or any other NSAIDs without your doctor's approval. In addition, consult your doctor if you are taking antihypertensives, steroids, anticoagulants, antibiotics, itraconazole or ketoconazole, plicamycin, penicillamine, valproic acid, phenytoin, cyclosporine, digitalis drugs, lithium, methotrexate, probenecid, triamterene, or zidovudine.

FOOD INTERACTIONS
No known food interactions.

DISEASE INTERACTIONS
Consult your doctor if you have any of the following: bleeding problems, gastrointestinal inflammation or ulcers, diabetes mellitus, systemic lupus erythematosus (SLE, lupus), anemia, asthma, epilepsy, Parkinson's disease, kidney stones, or a history of heart disease or alcohol abuse. Use of ketoprofen may cause complications in patients with liver or kidney disease, since these organs work together to remove the medication from the body.

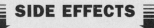 SIDE EFFECTS

SERIOUS
Shortness of breath or wheezing, with or without swelling of legs or other signs of heart failure; chest pain; peptic ulcer disease with vomiting of blood; black, tarry stools; decreasing kidney function. Call your doctor immediately.

COMMON
Nausea, vomiting, heartburn, diarrhea, constipation, headache, dizziness, sleepiness.

LESS COMMON
Ulcers or sores in mouth, depression, rashes or blistering of skin, ringing sound in the ears, unusual tingling or numbness of the hands or feet, seizures, blurred vision. Also elevated potassium levels, decreased blood counts; such problems can be detected by your doctor.

LOPERAMIDE HYDROCHLORIDE

Available in: Capsules, oral solution, tablets
Available as Generic? Yes
Drug Class: Antidiarrheal

▼ USAGE INFORMATION

WHY IT'S TAKEN
To treat diarrhea.

HOW IT WORKS
Loperamide relieves diarrhea by slowing the activity of the intestines.

▼ DOSAGE GUIDELINES

RANGE AND FREQUENCY
Capsules—Adults and teenagers: 4 mg after the first loose bowel movement, 2 mg after each subsequent loose bowel movement. Take no more than 16 mg every 24 hours. Children ages 8 to 12: 2 mg, 3 times a day. Children ages 6 to 8: 2 mg, 2 times a day. Oral solution—Adults and teenagers: 4 mg (4 teaspoons) after the first loose bowel movement, 2 mg after each subsequent loose bowel movement. No more than 8 mg every 24 hours. Children ages 9 to 11: 2 mg after the first loose bowel movement, 1 mg after each subsequent loose bowel movement. No more than 6 mg every 24 hours. Children ages 6 to 8: 2 mg after the first loose bowel movement, 1 mg after each subsequent loose bowel movement. No more than 4 mg every 24 hours. Tablets—Adults and teenagers: 4 mg after the first loose bowel movement, 1 mg after each subsequent loose bowel movement. No more than 8 mg every 24 hours. Children ages 9 to 11: 2 mg after the first loose bowel movement, 1 mg after each subsequent loose bowel movement. No more than 6 mg every 24 hours. Children ages 6 to 8: 2 mg after the first loose bowel movement, 1 mg after each subsequent loose bowel movement. No more than 4 mg every 24 hours.

ONSET OF EFFECT
Unknown.

DURATION OF ACTION
Up to 24 hours.

DIETARY ADVICE
Take it on an empty stomach (1 hour before or 2 hours after eating). A mild diet is recommended when recovering from diarrhea. Bananas, rice, applesauce, and plain toast are good choices. Be sure to drink plenty of fluids.

STORAGE
Store this medication in a tightly sealed container away from heat, moisture, and direct light.

MISSED DOSE
Skip the missed dose and resume your regular dosage schedule. Do not double the next dose.

STOPPING THE DRUG
You may stop taking the drug whenever you choose.

PROLONGED USE
Loperamide should not be used for more than 2 days unless directed otherwise by your doctor.

▼ PRECAUTIONS

Over 60: Diarrhea may easily lead to dehydration, especially in older patients, and loperamide may mask the effects of dehydration. When using loperamide, older persons should be sure to get plenty of fluids.

Driving and Hazardous Work: Avoid such activities until you determine how the medicine affects you.

Alcohol: Avoid alcohol.

Pregnancy: Discuss with your doctor the relative risks and benefits of using loperamide while pregnant.

Breast Feeding: It is not known whether loperamide passes into breast milk; caution is advised. Consult your doctor for specific advice.

Infants and Children: Do not give to children under 6 years of age unless otherwise directed by your doctor.

Special Concerns: During the first 24 hours, drink plenty of caffeine-free clear liquids like water, broth, ginger ale, and decaffeinated tea. During the second 24 hours, eat bland foods such as applesauce, bread, crackers, and oatmeal.

OVERDOSE
Symptoms: Constipation, central nervous system depression, gastrointestinal irritation.

What to Do: An overdose of loperamide is unlikely to be life-threatening. However, if someone takes a much larger dose than prescribed, call your doctor, emergency medical services (EMS), or the nearest poison control center.

▼ INTERACTIONS

DRUG INTERACTIONS
Consult your doctor for specific advice if you are taking antibiotics such as cephalosporin, erythromycin, and tetracycline; or any narcotic pain medication.

FOOD INTERACTIONS
Fruits, fried or spicy foods, bran, candy, and caffeine-containing beverages can make diarrhea worse.

DISEASE INTERACTIONS
Consult your doctor if you have an intestinal illness, severe colitis, or liver disease.

≡ SIDE EFFECTS ≡

▼ SERIOUS ▼
Bloating, skin rash, constipation, loss of appetite, stomach pains, nausea, vomiting. Call your doctor immediately.

COMMON
No common side effects are associated with loperamide.

LESS COMMON
Dizziness or drowsiness, dry mouth.

LOPERAMIDE/SIMETHICONE

Available in: Chewable tablet
Available as Generic? No
Drug Class: Antidiarrheal/antigas combination

▼ USAGE INFORMATION

WHY IT'S TAKEN
To treat diarrhea and to relieve bloating, pain, pressure, and cramps caused by excess gas in the stomach and intestines.

HOW IT WORKS
Loperamide eases diarrhea by slowing the activity of the intestines. Simethicone disperses and prevents the formation of gas bubbles in the gastrointestinal tract.

▼ DOSAGE GUIDELINES

RANGE AND FREQUENCY
Adults and teenagers: Chew 2 tablets and drink a full glass of water after the first loose stool. If needed, chew 1 tablet and drink more water after the next loose stool. Take no more than 4 tablets per day. Children ages 6 to 11: Chew 1 tablet after the first loose stool. If needed, chew half a tablet after the next loose stool. Children ages 9 to 11 (or weighing 60 to 95 lbs) should take no more than 3 tablets per day. Children ages 6 to 8 (or weighing 48 to 59 lbs) should take no more than 2 tablets per day. Follow each dose with plenty of clear liquids.

ONSET OF EFFECT
Unknown.

DURATION OF ACTION
Unknown.

DIETARY ADVICE
A mild diet is recommended when recovering from diarrhea. Bananas, rice, applesauce, and plain toast are good choices. Be sure to drink plenty of fluids.

STORAGE
Store in a tightly sealed container away from moisture, heat, and direct light.

MISSED DOSE
Not applicable, since the drug is taken only when necessary.

STOPPING THE DRUG
You may stop taking the drug whenever you choose.

PROLONGED USE
This drug should not be used for more than 2 days unless directed otherwise by your doctor.

▼ PRECAUTIONS

Over 60: Diarrhea may easily lead to dehydration, especially in older patients, and this drug may mask the symptoms of dehydration. When using this drug, older persons should be sure to get plenty of fluids.

Driving and Hazardous Work: No special precautions are necessary.

Alcohol: Avoid alcohol, as it may irritate the lining of the gastrointestinal tract and promote dehydration.

Pregnancy: Discuss with your doctor the relative risks and benefits of using this drug while pregnant.

Breast Feeding: This drug may pass into breast milk; caution is advised. Consult your doctor for specific advice.

Infants and Children: Not recommended for use by children younger than age 6 or who weigh less than 48 lbs.

Special Concerns: Chew the tablets thoroughly before swallowing for quicker and more complete relief. You should change position frequently and walk about to help eliminate gas. During the first 24 hours, drink plenty of caffeine-free clear liquids like water, broth, ginger ale, and decaffeinated tea. During the second 24 hours you may eat bland foods such as applesauce, bread, crackers, and oatmeal. Tell your doctor if you have diarrhea while on a low-sodium, low-sugar or other special diet. Do not smoke before meals.

OVERDOSE
Symptoms: Constipation, gastrointestinal irritation, drowsiness, confusion.

What to Do: An overdose of this drug is unlikely to be life-threatening. However, if someone takes a much larger dose than prescribed, call your doctor.

▼ INTERACTIONS

DRUG INTERACTIONS
Consult your doctor for specific advice if you are taking antibiotics such as cephalosporin, erythromycin, and tetracycline, or any narcotic pain medication.

FOOD INTERACTIONS
Fruits, fried or spicy foods, bran, candy, and caffeine-containing beverages can make diarrhea worse. Avoid any foods that increase gas formation. Chew your food slowly and thoroughly.

DISEASE INTERACTIONS
Do not use this drug if you have a high fever (over 101°F) or stools containing blood or mucus. Consult your physician before using this drug if you have an intestinal illness, severe colitis, or liver disease.

≣ SIDE EFFECTS ≣

SERIOUS
Skin rash, bloating, constipation, loss of appetite, stomach pain, nausea, vomiting. Call your doctor immediately.

COMMON
Expulsion of excess gas, causing belching and flatulence.

LESS COMMON
Dizziness or drowsiness, dry mouth.

MAGALDRATE

BRAND NAMES

Losopan, Riopan

Available in: Oral suspension
Available as Generic? Yes
Drug Class: Antacid

▼ USAGE INFORMATION

WHY IT'S TAKEN
To relieve symptoms of heartburn, acid indigestion, sour stomach, and gastroesophageal reflux. Also used to treat hyperacidity associated with peptic ulcers, gastritis, and esophagitis.

HOW IT WORKS
Magaldrate neutralizes stomach acid and reduces the action of pepsin, a digestive enzyme. This provides symptomatic relief from excess stomach acid.

▼ DOSAGE GUIDELINES

RANGE AND FREQUENCY
Adults: 540 to 1,080 mg (5 to 10 ml). Children: 5 to 10 mg. Take it between meals and at bedtime.

ONSET OF EFFECT
Within 20 minutes.

DURATION OF ACTION
20 to 60 minutes in fasting patients; 3 hours when taken after meals.

DIETARY ADVICE
Eat a balanced diet.

STORAGE
Store in a tightly sealed container away from moisture, heat, and direct light.

MISSED DOSE
Take it as soon as you remember. If it is near the time for the next dose, skip the missed dose and resume your regular dosage schedule. Do not double the next dose.

STOPPING THE DRUG
Take as directed for the full treatment period.

PROLONGED USE
Do not take magaldrate for more than 2 weeks unless your doctor advises you to do otherwise.

≡ SIDE EFFECTS ≡

SERIOUS
Severe and continuing constipation, dizziness, lightheadedness, and heartbeat irregularities. Bone loss (osteomalacia) may occur, especially with prolonged use in dialysis patients. Hypophosphatemia (too little phosphate in the blood) may occur with prolonged use and a low-phosphate diet; symptoms include bone pain, fractures (due to bone loss), muscle weakness, loss of appetite, mood changes, a general feeling of discomfort, swelling of the wrists and ankles, unusual weight loss, and anemia (decreased number of red blood cells; symptoms include weakness and fatigue). Call your doctor immediately.

COMMON
Chalky taste.

LESS COMMON
Increased thirst, speckling or whitish color of stools, stomach cramps, diarrhea, mild constipation.

▼ PRECAUTIONS

Over 60: Constipation and intestinal trouble are more common in older persons. Older patients who have or who are at high risk for osteoporosis or other bone disorders should avoid frequent use of magaldrate.

Driving and Hazardous Work: No special precautions.

Alcohol: Avoid alcohol.

Pregnancy: Adequate studies have not been done. Before taking magaldrate, tell your doctor if you are pregnant or plan to become pregnant.

Breast Feeding: Magaldrate may pass into breast milk but has not been reported to cause problems in nursing babies. Consult your doctor for advice.

Infants and Children: Do not give antacids and other magnesium-containing medicines to young children unless prescribed by a physician.

Special Concerns: Use over-the-counter antacids only occasionally unless otherwise directed by your doctor. Persistent heartburn not readily relieved by antacids may be signaling a heart attack or other serious disorder. Seek medical help promptly.

OVERDOSE
Symptoms: Diarrhea, nausea, vomiting, constipation, confusion, palpitations, weakness, fatigue, bone pain, stupor.

What to Do: An overdose of magaldrate is unlikely to be life-threatening. However, if someone takes a much larger dose than prescribed, call your doctor, emergency medical services (EMS), or the nearest poison control center.

▼ INTERACTIONS

DRUG INTERACTIONS
Magaldrate and other magnesium-containing antacids may interact with vitamin D (including calcitediol and calcitriol), and may decrease the effectiveness of pancrelipase. Note that other medications may lose their effectiveness when taken within 1 hour of antacids. Consult your doctor for specific advice if you are taking amphetamines, bisacodyl, cellulose sodium phosphate, citrates, chenodiol, digoxin, enteric-coated medications, fluoroquinolones, isoniazid, ketoconazole, mecamylamine, methenamine, nitrofurantoin, penicillamine, phosphates, sodium polystyrene sulfonate resin, tetracyclines, or quinidine,

FOOD INTERACTIONS
No known food interactions.

DISEASE INTERACTIONS
Do not take magaldrate if you have any symptoms of appendicitis or an inflamed bowel (abdominal pain, cramps, soreness, bloating, nausea, and vomiting). Magaldrate is not recommended for Alzheimer's patients. Consult your doctor if you have any of the following: broken bones, colitis, diarrhea, intestinal blockage or bleeding, colostomy or ileostomy, edema, hypophosphatemia, heart disease, liver disease, toxemia of pregnancy, or kidney disease.

MAGNESIUM CITRATE

BRAND NAMES
Citrate of Magnesia,
Citro-Nesia, Citroma

Available in: Oral solution
Available as Generic? Yes
Drug Class: Hyperosmotic laxative

▼ USAGE INFORMATION

WHY IT'S TAKEN
To treat short-term constipation and for rapid emptying of the colon for rectal and bowel examinations.

HOW IT WORKS
Magnesium citrate attracts and retains water in the intestine, softening stools and inducing the urge to defecate.

▼ DOSAGE GUIDELINES

RANGE AND FREQUENCY
Adults and teenagers: 11 to 25 g daily in 1 or more doses. Children ages 6 to 12: 5.5 to 12.5 g daily in 1 or more doses.

ONSET OF EFFECT
30 minutes to 3 hours.

DURATION OF ACTION
Variable.

DIETARY ADVICE
Take it on an empty stomach with a full glass of cold water or juice.

STORAGE
Store in a tightly sealed container away from moisture, heat, and direct light.

MISSED DOSE
If you are taking this drug on a fixed schedule, take the missed dose as soon as you remember. If it is near the time for the next dose, skip the missed dose and resume your regular dosage schedule. Do not double the next dose.

STOPPING THE DRUG
Take it as prescribed for the full treatment period. However, you may stop taking the drug if you are feeling better before the scheduled end of the therapy.

PROLONGED USE
Magnesium citrate is intended for short-term therapy only.

▼ PRECAUTIONS

Over 60: No special problems are expected.

Driving and Hazardous Work: This medication should not impair your ability to perform such tasks safely.

Alcohol: Avoid alcohol.

Pregnancy: Pregnant women with impaired kidney function should avoid taking magnesium citrate.

Breast Feeding: Magnesium citrate may pass into breast milk; caution is advised. Consult your doctor for advice.

Infants and Children: Do not give magnesium citrate and other laxatives to children under 6 years of age unless prescribed by a doctor.

Special Concerns: Chilling the medication, taking it with ice, or following it with citrus fruit juice or citrus-flavored carbonated beverages may make it more palatable. Remember that chronic use of magnesium citrate or any laxative can lead to laxative dependence. You should consume adequate amounts of fiber in your diet, like bran, whole-grain cereals, fruit, and vegetables. Magnesium citrate should be taken on a schedule that doesn't interfere with activities or sleep, as it produces watery stools in 3 to 6 hours. It should not be taken within 2 hours of taking other medications.

OVERDOSE
Symptoms: Severe or protracted diarrhea.

What to Do: An overdose of magnesium citrate is unlikely to be life-threatening. However, if someone takes a much larger dose than prescribed, call your doctor, emergency medical services (EMS), or the nearest poison control center right away.

▼ INTERACTIONS

DRUG INTERACTIONS
Consult your doctor for specific advice if you are taking cellulose sodium phosphate; other magnesium-containing medications such as antacids; other laxatives; sodium polystyrene sulfonate; and oral tetracycline antibiotics.

FOOD INTERACTIONS
No known food interactions.

DISEASE INTERACTIONS
Caution is advised when taking magnesium citrate. Consult your doctor if you have kidney problems, symptoms of appendicitis (abdominal pain, nausea, vomiting), heart damage, intestinal obstruction or perforation, heart block, or rectal fissures.

≡ SIDE EFFECTS ≡

SERIOUS
Confusion, dizziness or lightheadedness, intestinal blockage, skin rash or itching, difficulty swallowing. Call your doctor immediately.

COMMON
Cramping, diarrhea, gas, increased thirst.

LESS COMMON
Sweating, weakness.

MAGNESIUM OXIDE

Available in: Capsules, tablets
Available as Generic? Yes
Drug Class: Antacid

▼ USAGE INFORMATION

WHY IT'S TAKEN
To treat low magnesium in the blood (hypomagnesemia). Also used to replace or prevent magnesium loss due to other medications or conditions. It is used as an antacid to relieve heartburn, sour stomach, and acid indigestion.

HOW IT WORKS
Magnesium oxide neutralizes stomach acid and reduces the action of pepsin, a digestive enzyme. This provides symptomatic relief from excess stomach acid and heartburn.

▼ DOSAGE GUIDELINES

RANGE AND FREQUENCY
Capsules: 140 mg, 3 to 4 times a day. Tablets: 400 to 800 mg a day in evenly divided doses.

ONSET OF EFFECT
Within 20 minutes.

DURATION OF ACTION
For 20 minutes in fasting patients; 3 hours when taken after meals.

DIETARY ADVICE
Take this medication at least 1 hour after meals.

STORAGE
Store in a tightly sealed container away from moisture, heat, and direct light.

MISSED DOSE
Take it as soon as you remember. If it is near the time for the next dose, skip the missed dose and resume your regular dosage schedule. Do not double the next dose.

STOPPING THE DRUG
Take it as prescribed for the full treatment period. However, when magnesium oxide is used as an antacid, it may be taken as needed.

PROLONGED USE
You should see your doctor regularly for tests and examinations if you must take this drug for a prolonged period.

▼ PRECAUTIONS

Over 60: Adverse reactions may be more likely and more severe.

Driving and Hazardous Work: Do not drive or engage in hazardous work until you determine how the medicine affects you.

Alcohol: Avoid alcohol.

Pregnancy: Adequate studies have not been done. Be sure to tell your doctor if you are pregnant or planning to become pregnant.

Breast Feeding: Magnesium oxide may pass into breast milk; consult your doctor for advice.

Infants and Children: Not recommended for use by children under 6 unless prescribed by a doctor.

Special Concerns: Using magnesium oxide in large amounts or for prolonged periods may have a laxative effect; the drug should not be used regularly for this purpose. In general, do not take other medicines within 2 hours of taking magnesium-containing antacids. Upper abdominal pain or heartburn not readily relieved by antacids may be signaling a heart attack or other serious disorder. In such cases, seek medical help promptly.

OVERDOSE
Symptoms: Diarrhea, bloating, change in mental state, muscle pain or twitching, slowed or shallow breathing, coma.

What to Do: An overdose of magnesium oxide is unlikely to be life-threatening. However, if someone takes a much larger dose than prescribed, call your doctor, emergency medical services (EMS), or the nearest poison control center immediately.

▼ INTERACTIONS

DRUG INTERACTIONS
Consult your doctor if you are taking fluoroquinolones, ketoconazole, methenamine, mecamylamine, sodium polystyrene sulfonate, tetracyclines, urinary acidifiers, digitalis drugs, misoprostol, pancrelipase, iron salts, phosphates, salicylates, or vitamin D (including calcifediol and calcitriol). Also, certain medications may lose their effectiveness or cause unexpected side effects when taken within 2 hours of magnesium oxide. These include enteric-coated medicines, folic acid, penicillamine, phenothiazines, and phenytoin. Take at least 2 hours apart (and 3 hours before or after phenytoin).

FOOD INTERACTIONS
No known food interactions.

DISEASE INTERACTIONS
Do not take magnesium oxide if you have any symptoms of appendicitis or an inflamed bowel (abdominal pain, cramps, soreness, bloating, nausea, and vomiting). Magnesium-containing antacids should not be taken by patients with kidney disease. Consult your doctor if you have any of the following: bone fractures, colitis, severe and continuing constipation, hemorrhoids, intestinal or rectal bleeding, a colostomy or ileostomy, persistent diarrhea, edema, heart disease, liver disease, preeclampsia, sarcoidosis, or underactive parathyroid glands.

≡ SIDE EFFECTS ≡

SERIOUS
Dizziness, lightheadedness, continuing feeling of discomfort, irregular heartbeat, loss of appetite, mental or mood changes, muscle weakness, unusual fatigue or weakness, unusual weight loss. Call your doctor immediately.

COMMON
Chalky taste, laxative effect.

LESS COMMON
Diarrhea, increased thirst, speckling or discoloration of stools, stomach cramps, nausea or vomiting, elevated magnesium in the blood (detectable by your doctor).

MAGNESIUM SULFATE

Available in: Crystals, tablets
Available as Generic? Yes
Drug Class: Laxative/dietary supplement

▼ USAGE INFORMATION

WHY IT'S TAKEN
Magnesium sulfate is used to evacuate the bowel before surgery, and as a dietary supplement for people with a magnesium deficiency due to illness or as a result of the use of certain medications.

HOW IT WORKS
As a laxative, magnesium sulfate attracts and retains water in the intestine, softening stools and inducing the urge to defecate.

▼ DOSAGE GUIDELINES

RANGE AND FREQUENCY
As a laxative—Adults and teenagers: 10 to 30 g daily in 1 or more doses. Children ages 6 to 12: 5 to 10 g daily in 1 or more doses. To treat magnesium deficiency—The dose is determined by your doctor according to the severity of the deficiency.

ONSET OF EFFECT
Within 30 minutes to 3 hours.

DURATION OF ACTION
Variable.

DIETARY ADVICE
Take it on an empty stomach with a full glass of cold water or juice.

STORAGE
Store in a tightly sealed container away from heat, moisture, and direct light.

MISSED DOSE
If you are taking this drug on a fixed schedule, take the missed dose as soon as you remember. If it is near the time for the next dose, skip the missed dose and resume your regular dosage schedule. Do not double the next dose.

STOPPING THE DRUG
You should not take magnesium sulfate for more than 1 week unless your physician prescribes its continued use.

PROLONGED USE
You should see your doctor regularly for tests and examinations if you must take this drug for a prolonged period.

▼ PRECAUTIONS

Over 60: No special problems are expected.

≣ SIDE EFFECTS ≣

▼ SERIOUS ▼
Abdominal cramps, nausea, diarrhea. Call your doctor immediately.

COMMON
There are no common side effects associated with the use of magnesium sulfate.

LESS COMMON
There are no less-common side effects associated with the use of magnesium sulfate.

Driving and Hazardous Work: The use of magnesium sulfate should not impair your ability to perform such tasks safely.

Alcohol: Avoid alcohol.

Pregnancy: Magnesium sulfate is used as a treatment, in the hospital only, for certain symptoms of preeclampsia. If necessary, pregnant women can take magnesium sulfate as a dietary supplement.

Breast Feeding: Magnesium sulfate passes into breast milk; caution is advised. Consult your doctor for advice.

Infants and Children: Magnesium sulfate and other laxatives should not be given to children under 6 years of age unless prescribed by your pediatrician.

Special Concerns: Taking magnesium sulfate with ice or following it with citrus fruit juice or a citrus-flavored carbonated beverage may make it more palatable. Remember that chronic use of magnesium sulfate or any laxative can lead to laxative dependence. Consume adequate amounts of fiber in your diet, such as bran, fruit, whole-grain cereals, and vegetables. It should be taken on a schedule that does not interfere with activities or sleep, as it produces watery stools within 3 to 6 hours. It should not be taken within 2 hours of taking other drugs.

OVERDOSE
Symptoms: Blurred or double vision, dizziness or fainting, severe drowsiness, increased or decreased urination, slow heartbeat, trouble breathing.

What to Do: Call your doctor, emergency medical services (EMS), or the nearest poison control center immediately.

▼ INTERACTIONS

DRUG INTERACTIONS
Consult your doctor for specific advice if you are taking oral tetracycline, other preparations containing magnesium, cellulose sodium phosphate, sodium polystyrene sulfonate, or digitalis drugs.

FOOD INTERACTIONS
No known food interactions.

DISEASE INTERACTIONS
Use caution when taking magnesium sulfate. Consult your doctor if you have any of the following: myasthenia gravis, severe kidney disease, heart blockage, intestinal obstruction or perforation, or any respiratory disease.

MECLIZINE

Available in: Capsules, tablets, chewable tablets
Available as Generic? Yes
Drug Class: Antiemetic; antivertigo agent

▼ USAGE INFORMATION

WHY IT'S TAKEN
To treat and prevent nausea, vomiting, and dizziness caused by motion sickness, as well as to treat vertigo (dizziness) associated with other medical problems.

HOW IT WORKS
Meclizine acts on the brain centers that control nausea, vomiting, and dizziness.

▼ DOSAGE GUIDELINES

RANGE AND FREQUENCY
To prevent and treat motion sickness—Adults and teenagers: 25 to 50 mg, 1 hour before travel; the dose may be repeated every 24 hours. To prevent and treat vertigo—Adults and teenagers: 25 to 100 mg a day as needed, in divided doses.

ONSET OF EFFECT
Within 1 hour.

DURATION OF ACTION
Up to 24 hours.

DIETARY ADVICE
Can be taken with food.

STORAGE
Store in a tightly sealed container protected from heat, moisture, and direct light.

MISSED DOSE
Take it as soon as you remember. If it is near the time for the next dose, skip the missed dose and resume your regular dosage schedule. Do not double the next dose.

STOPPING THE DRUG
Take it as prescribed for the full treatment period. However, you may stop taking the medication if you are feeling better before the scheduled end of therapy.

PROLONGED USE
See your doctor regularly for tests and examinations if you must use this drug for a prolonged period.

▼ PRECAUTIONS

Over 60: Adverse reactions may be more likely and more severe in older patients.

Driving and Hazardous Work: Do not drive or engage in hazardous work until you determine how the medicine affects you.

Alcohol: Avoid alcohol when using this medication.

Pregnancy: Adequate human studies have not been completed. Before taking meclizine, tell your doctor if you are pregnant or plan to become pregnant.

Breast Feeding: Meclizine may pass into breast milk but has not been reported to cause problems in nursing babies. It may reduce the flow of breast milk. Consult your doctor for advice.

Infants and Children: Meclizine is not recommended for use by children under the age of 12.

Special Concerns: If dry mouth occurs, use sugarless candy or gum or bits of ice for temporary relief. If constipation occurs, a high-fiber diet and drinking plenty of fluids can help relieve the problem. Meclizine can cause false-negative results in allergy skin testing.

OVERDOSE
Symptoms: Extreme excitability, seizures, drowsiness, hallucinations.

What to Do: Call your doctor, emergency medical services (EMS), or the nearest poison control center immediately.

▼ INTERACTIONS

DRUG INTERACTIONS
Consult your doctor for specific advice if you are taking medications that can depress the central nervous system, such as tranquilizers, sleep medications, antihistamines, medicines for hay fever, prescription pain medicines, or muscle relaxants, or if you are taking any additional OTC medication.

FOOD INTERACTIONS
No known food interactions.

DISEASE INTERACTIONS
Caution is advised when taking meclizine. Consult your doctor if you have any of the following: urinary tract blockage, glaucoma, asthma, bronchitis, emphysema, any other chronic lung disease, enlarged prostate, heart failure, or intestinal blockage.

≣ SIDE EFFECTS ≣

▼ SERIOUS ▼
No serious side effects are associated with the use of meclizine.

COMMON
Drowsiness.

LESS COMMON
Blurred or double vision; upset stomach; constipation or diarrhea; insomnia; painful or difficult urination; dizziness; dry mouth, nose, and throat; headache; loss of appetite; fast heartbeat; nervousness; restlessness; skin rash.

MICONAZOLE

Available in: Vaginal cream and suppositories
Available as Generic? Yes
Drug Class: Antifungal

▼ USAGE INFORMATION

WHY IT'S TAKEN
To treat severe fungal infections, particularly vaginal yeast infections.

HOW IT WORKS
Miconazole prevents fungal organisms from producing vital substances required for growth and function. This medication is effective only for infections caused by fungal organisms. It will not be effective against bacterial or viral infections.

▼ DOSAGE GUIDELINES

RANGE AND FREQUENCY
Adults and teenagers—Vaginal cream: At bedtime, insert into the vagina 1 applicatorful for 7 to 14 nights. Vaginal suppositories: At bedtime, insert one 100-mg suppository into the vagina for 7 nights, or one 200-mg or one 400-mg suppository for 3 nights.

ONSET OF EFFECT
Unknown.

DURATION OF ACTION
Unknown.

DIETARY ADVICE
No special restrictions.

STORAGE
Store in a tightly sealed container away from moisture, heat, and direct light. Refrigerate the suppositories, and do not allow the medication to freeze.

MISSED DOSE
Take it as soon as you remember. This will help keep a constant level of medication in your system. If it is near the time for the next dose, skip the missed dose and resume your regular dosage schedule. Do not double the next dose.

STOPPING THE DRUG
Take as directed for the full treatment period, even if you begin to feel better before the scheduled end of therapy. Stopping prematurely increases the risk of reinfection. Some fungal infections take many months to clear up, and some may require continuous treatment.

PROLONGED USE
Therapy with this medication may require months. Prolonged use may increase the risk of adverse effects.

▼ PRECAUTIONS

Over 60: Adverse reactions may be more likely and more severe in older patients.

Driving and Hazardous Work: Do not drive or engage in hazardous work until you determine how the medicine affects you.

Alcohol: Avoid alcohol.

Pregnancy: Adequate studies of miconazole use during pregnancy have not been done. Consult your doctor for advice if you are pregnant or are planning to become pregnant.

Breast Feeding: Miconazole passes into breast milk; caution is advised. Consult your doctor for advice.

Infants and Children: Not recommended for use by children under age 1.

Special Concerns: Sanitary napkins should be used to prevent staining of clothing. The affected area should be kept cool and dry. Do not sit for a long time in a wet bathing suit. Avoid feminine hygiene sprays. Wash daily with unscented soap and dry thoroughly with a clean towel. Tampons should not be used during therapy. The patient's sexual partner should wear a condom during intercourse. Do not stop using this medicine during your menstrual period. After urination or a bowel movement, cleanse by wiping the area from front to back to prevent reinfection.

OVERDOSE
Symptoms: An overdose with miconazole is unlikely.

What to Do: Emergency instructions not applicable.

▼ INTERACTIONS

DRUG INTERACTIONS
Tell your doctor if you are using any other vaginal prescription or OTC medicine when using the vaginal forms. Do not take medications containing alcohol, such as cough syrups, elixirs, and tonics. Consult your doctor for specific advice if you are taking cyclosporine, phenytoin, or warfarin.

FOOD INTERACTIONS
No known food interactions.

DISEASE INTERACTIONS
Consult your doctor if you have a history of alcohol abuse. Use of miconazole can cause complications in patients with liver or kidney disease, since these organs work together to remove the medication from the body.

≡ SIDE EFFECTS ≡
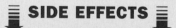

SERIOUS
Skin rash or itching; fever or chills; pain at site of injection; vaginal burning, itching, discharge, or irritation not present prior to treatment. Call your doctor immediately.

COMMON
No common side effects are associated with miconazole.

LESS COMMON
Diarrhea, nausea, vomiting, constipation, dizziness, headache, redness or flushing of skin, stomach cramps or pain, burning or irritation of sexual partner's penis.

MILK OF MAGNESIA (MAGNESIA; MAGNESIUM HYDROXIDE)

Available in: Oral suspension, chewable tablets
Available as Generic? Yes
Drug Class: Antacid/hyperosmotic laxative

▼ USAGE INFORMATION

WHY IT'S TAKEN
To relieve symptoms of upset stomach; sometimes used also for short-term treatment of constipation.

HOW IT WORKS
As an antacid, milk of magnesia neutralizes stomach acid. As a laxative, it attracts and retains water in the intestine, increasing intestinal movement (peristalsis) and inducing the urge to defecate.

▼ DOSAGE GUIDELINES

RANGE AND FREQUENCY
As an antacid—Adults and teenagers. 5 to 15 ml of liquid form or 650 mg to 1.3 g of tablets 3 or 4 times a day. To relieve constipation—Adults and teenagers: 2.4 to 4.8 g (30 to 60 ml) daily in 1 or more doses. Children ages 6 to 12: 1.2 to 2.4 g (15 to 30 ml) daily in 1 or more doses.

ONSET OF EFFECT
30 minutes to 3 hours.

DURATION OF ACTION
Variable.

DIETARY ADVICE
Take it 1 to 3 hours after meals or at bedtime with a full glass of water.

STORAGE
Store milk of magnesia in a tightly sealed container away from heat, moisture, and direct light.

MISSED DOSE
Take it as soon as you remember. If it is near the time for the next dose, skip the missed dose and resume your regular dosage schedule. Do not double the next dose.

STOPPING THE DRUG
You may stop taking the drug whenever you choose.

PROLONGED USE
Do not take milk of magnesia for more than 2 weeks unless your doctor prescribes it.

▼ PRECAUTIONS

Over 60: No special advice.

Driving and Hazardous Work: This medicine should not impair your ability to perform such tasks safely.

Alcohol: Avoid alcohol.

Pregnancy: Extensive human studies have not been done. There have been reports of side effects in babies whose mothers took high doses of antacids for a long time during pregnancy. Before you take milk of magnesia, consult your doctor if you are pregnant or if you plan to become pregnant.

Breast Feeding: Milk of magnesia may pass into breast milk but has not been reported to cause problems in nursing babies. Consult your doctor for advice.

Infants and Children: Antacids and other medications containing magnesium should not be given to children under age 6 unless prescribed by a doctor.

Special Concerns: Take milk of magnesia on a schedule that does not interfere with activities or sleep, as it produces watery stools in 3 to 6 hours. Remember that frequent or protracted use can lead to laxative dependence. Do not take milk of magnesia within 2 hours of taking other medications. Before swallowing, chew tablets well to allow the medicine to work more quickly and effectively.

OVERDOSE

Symptoms: Severe or protracted diarrhea, painful or difficult urination, muscle weakness, continuing loss of appetite, irregular heartbeat, difficulty breathing.

What to Do: An overdose of milk of magnesia is unlikely to be life threatening. However, if someone takes a much larger dose than prescribed, call your doctor, emergency medical services (EMS), or the nearest poison control center immediately.

▼ INTERACTIONS

DRUG INTERACTIONS
Consult your physician for specific advice if you are taking other antacids or laxatives, or any of the following medications: cellulose sodium phosphate, fluoroquinolones, isoniazid, ketoconazole, sodium polystyrene sulfonate resin, methenamine, mecamylamine, salicylates, or tetracyclines.

FOOD INTERACTIONS
None are known.

DISEASE INTERACTIONS
Do not use this medication if you have any symptoms of appendicitis or inflamed bowel such as lower abdominal or stomach pain, nausea or vomiting, cramping, soreness, or bloating. Consult your physician if you have any of the following: broken bones, colitis, hemorrhoids, intestinal blockage or bleeding, a recent colostomy or ileostomy, swelling of feet or lower legs, heart disease, toxemia of pregnancy, liver disease, or kidney disease.

≡ SIDE EFFECTS ≡

SERIOUS
Dizziness or lightheadedness, continuing feeling of discomfort, irregular heartbeat, loss of appetite, mood or mental changes, muscle weakness, unusual fatigue, unusual weight loss, rectal bleeding. Call your doctor immediately.

COMMON
Nausea, diarrhea.

LESS COMMON
Increased thirst, speckling or whitish color of stools, abdominal cramps.

MINOXIDIL TOPICAL

Rogaine

Available in: Topical solution
Available as Generic? Yes
Drug Class: Hair growth stimulant

▼ USAGE INFORMATION

WHY IT'S TAKEN
Minoxidil topical solution is prescribed to stimulate hair growth in men and women with the type of baldness known as androgenetic alopecia, a condition which is popularly known as male pattern baldness or female pattern baldness.

HOW IT WORKS
It is not known how minoxidil works. Although it increases the flow of blood, nutrients, and other important substances to hair follicles, other or additional poorly understood actions are believed responsible for hair growth.

▼ DOSAGE GUIDELINES

RANGE AND FREQUENCY
Adults: Apply 1 ml regardless of the size of the balding area under treatment.

ONSET OF EFFECT
At least 4 months with twice daily therapy.

DURATION OF ACTION
New hair resulting from minoxidil treatments will likely be lost approximately 3 to 4 months following the discontinuation of the medication.

DIETARY ADVICE
No special restrictions.

STORAGE
Store in a tightly sealed container away from heat and direct light. Keep away from moisture and extremes in temperature.

MISSED DOSE
Apply it as soon as you remember. If it is near the time for the next dose, skip the missed dose and resume your regular dosage schedule. Do not double the next dose.

STOPPING THE DRUG
Use it until you are able to assess changes, if any, in hair growth and cosmetic appearance. This may take at least 4 months. If you decide to abandon efforts to achieve hair regrowth, you may stop the medication at any time.

PROLONGED USE
Ongoing therapy with this medication is required for continued results. Prolonged use may increase the risk of undesirable side effects.

▼ PRECAUTIONS

Over 60: Adverse reactions may be more likely and more severe in older patients.

Driving and Hazardous Work: Do not drive or engage in hazardous work until you determine how the medicine affects you.

Alcohol: No special warnings.

Pregnancy: Avoid or discontinue topical minoxidil if you are pregnant or trying to become pregnant. Consult your physician.

Breast Feeding: Minoxidil passes into breast milk; do not use it while nursing.

Infants and Children: Not recommended for children.

Special Concerns: Anyone with a history of allergy to minoxidil or other components of the product should not use this medication. Minoxidil has potentially serious side effects if absorbed in large amounts into the body. Persons with a history of heart disease should consult their doctor before using this product. Do not apply to irritated, blistered, bleeding, or broken skin. Do not use more than the recommended dose, and do not apply it more frequently than twice a day. Do not use hairdryers to accelerate drying of the medication.

OVERDOSE
Symptoms: Symptoms are similar to those listed under serious side effects: rapid pulse; weakness, dizziness, or a lightheaded feeling; chest pain.

What to Do: If the above symptoms occur or someone ingests the medication, call your doctor, emergency medical services (EMS), or the nearest poison control center immediately.

▼ INTERACTIONS

DRUG INTERACTIONS
Consult your doctor for specific advice if you are taking oral minoxidil, steroids, petrolatum, or acne preparations such as tretinoin. Any person using heart or blood pressure medications should discuss minoxidil use with their doctor before starting treatment.

FOOD INTERACTIONS
No known food interactions.

DISEASE INTERACTIONS
Consult your doctor if you have any disorders affecting your skin or scalp, including rashes, sunburn, or other types of skin eruption or inflammation; heart disease; or high blood pressure.

≡ SIDE EFFECTS ≡

SERIOUS
Rapid pulse; weakness, dizziness, or lightheaded feeling; chest pain. Notify your doctor immediately. If chest pain is present, call emergency medical services (EMS).

COMMON
Burning, tingling, or mild redness of scalp at application site; mild dryness or flaking of skin; itching.

LESS COMMON
Significant irritation or allergy with redness, itching, flaking, or rash. Tingling of hands or feet; water retention (swelling of face, hands, fingers, or legs); flushing; headache. Stop the drug and notify your doctor immediately.

NAFARELIN ACETATE

Available in: Nasal spray
Available as Generic? No
Drug Class: Gonadotropin-releasing hormone

▼ USAGE INFORMATION

WHY IT'S TAKEN
To relieve the pain and dis-comfort of endometriosis.

HOW IT WORKS
Nafarelin decreases the pro-duction of estrogen by the ovaries. Reduced blood estro-gen levels lead to shrinking of endometrial tissue (uterine lining), which eases flare-ups of endometriosis.

▼ DOSAGE GUIDELINES

RANGE AND FREQUENCY
One spray of 200 micrograms into 1 nostril in the morning and 1 spray into the other nostril in the evening, begin-ning on day 2, 3, or 4 of the menstrual period.

ONSET OF EFFECT
After 4 weeks.

DURATION OF ACTION
3 to 6 months.

DIETARY ADVICE
No special restrictions.

STORAGE
Store container upright away from heat and direct light.

MISSED DOSE
Take it as soon as you remember. However, if it is near the time for the next dose, skip the missed dose and resume your regular dosage schedule. Do not double the next dose.

STOPPING THE DRUG
The decision to stop taking the drug should be made by your doctor.

PROLONGED USE
Your doctor should check your progress regularly during prolonged use.

▼ PRECAUTIONS

Over 60: This medicine is generally not used by older patients.

Driving and Hazardous Work: The use of nafarelin should not impair your ability to perform such tasks safely.

Alcohol: Avoid alcohol.

Pregnancy: Nafarelin is not recommended during preg-nancy. When taking the drug, women should use nonhor-monal contraception (that is, methods other than birth control pills). If you think you are pregnant, stop taking the medicine and call your doctor right away.

Breast Feeding: Nafarelin may pass into breast milk; caution is advised. Consult your doctor for advice.

Infants and Children: This drug is not recommended for use by children under the age of puberty.

Special Concerns: Tell your doctor if you smoke ciga-rettes or consume a lot of alcohol or caffeine. When using a new bottle of nafarelin spray, point the bottle away from you and pump about 7 times to prime it. Each time you use the spray, wipe the tip with a clean tissue or cloth. Every 3 or 4 days, rinse the tip with warm water and wipe the tip for about 15 seconds, then dry. To take a dose of nafarelin, first blow your nose gently. Hold your head forward a little, put the spray tip in the nostril, and aim for the back. Close the other nostril by pressing with 1 finger. After the spray, tilt your head back for a few sec-onds. Do not blow your nose.

OVERDOSE
Symptoms: No specific ones have been reported.

What to Do: An overdose of nafarelin is unlikely to be life-threatening. However, if someone takes a much larger dose than is recommended, call your doctor, emergency medical services (EMS), or the nearest poison control center immediately.

▼ INTERACTIONS

DRUG INTERACTIONS
Consult your doctor for spe-cific advice if you are taking any nasal spray decongestant, adrenocorticoids, or anticon-vulsant medication.

FOOD INTERACTIONS
No known food interactions.

DISEASE INTERACTIONS
Caution is advised when tak-ing nafarelin. Consult your doctor if you have any menstrual disorder.

≡ SIDE EFFECTS ≡

SERIOUS
Vaginal bleeding between menstrual periods; longer or heavier menstrual periods; shortness of breath, chest pain, joint pain, and hives caused by an allergic reaction; bloat-ing or tenderness of the lower abdomen; unexpected or excess flow of milk. Call your doctor immediately.

COMMON
Acne, decreased sex drive, dryness of vagina, hot flashes, pain during intercourse, decreased breast size, palpitations, oily skin, cessation of menstrual periods.

LESS COMMON
Breast pain, headache, runny nose, mental depression, mood swings, rash, weight changes.

NAPROXEN

Available in: Tablets, oral suspension, gelcaps
Available as Generic? Yes
Drug Class: Nonsteroidal anti-inflammatory drug (NSAID)

▼ USAGE INFORMATION

WHY IT'S TAKEN
To relieve minor pain or inflammation associated with headaches, the common cold, toothache, muscle aches, backache, arthritis, gout, tendinitis, bursitis, or menstrual cramps; also, to reduce fever. When patients fail to respond to one NSAID, several others may be tried.

HOW IT WORKS
NSAIDs work by interfering with the formation of prostaglandins, naturally occurring substances in the body that cause inflammation and make nerves more sensitive to pain impulses. NSAIDs also have other modes of action that are less well understood.

▼ DOSAGE GUIDELINES

RANGE AND FREQUENCY
Adults: 440 to 1,500 mg daily. Maximum dose is 1,500 mg a day, taken in 2 to 3 evenly divided doses.

ONSET OF EFFECT
Rapid; relieves pain within 1 hour. However, it may take up to 2 weeks to suppress inflammation.

DURATION OF ACTION
Up to 12 hours.

DIETARY ADVICE
Take with food; maintain your usual food and fluid intake.

STORAGE
Store tablets in a tightly sealed container away from heat, moisture, and direct light. Store oral suspension in refrigerator, but do not freeze.

MISSED DOSE
Take it as soon as you remember. However, if it is near the time for the next dose, skip the missed dose and resume your regular dosage schedule. Do not double the next dose.

STOPPING THE DRUG
If you are taking this drug by prescription, do not stop taking it without first consulting your doctor.

PROLONGED USE
Prolonged use can cause such gastrointestinal problems as ulceration and bleeding, kidney dysfunction, and liver inflammation. Consult your doctor about the need for medical examinations and lab studies.

▼ PRECAUTIONS

Over 60: Because of the potentially greater consequences of gastrointestinal side effects, the dose of NSAIDs for older patients, especially those over age 70, is often cut in half.

Driving and Hazardous Work: Avoid such activities until you determine how the medication affects you.

Alcohol: Avoid alcohol when taking this drug; the combination of naproxen and alcoholic beverages can be highly toxic to the liver.

Pregnancy: Avoid this drug if you are pregnant or plan to become pregnant.

Breast Feeding: Naproxen passes into breast milk; avoid use while nursing.

Infants and Children: Naproxen may be used in exceptional circumstances; consult your pediatrician for advice.

Special Concerns: Because NSAIDs can interfere with blood coagulation, this drug should be stopped at least 3 days prior to any surgery.

OVERDOSE

Symptoms: Severe nausea, vomiting, headache, confusion, seizures.

What to Do: Call your doctor, emergency medical services (EMS), or the nearest poison control center immediately.

▼ INTERACTIONS

DRUG INTERACTIONS
Do not take this drug with aspirin or any other NSAIDs without your doctor's approval. In addition, consult your doctor if you are taking antihypertensives, steroids, anticoagulants, antibiotics, itraconazole or ketoconazole, plicamycin, penicillamine, valproic acid, phenytoin, cyclosporine, digitalis drugs, lithium, methotrexate, probenecid, triamterene, or zidovudine.

FOOD INTERACTIONS
No known food interactions.

DISEASE INTERACTIONS
Consult your doctor if you have any of the following: bleeding problems, inflammation or ulcers of the stomach and intestines, diabetes mellitus, systemic lupus erythematosus (SLE, lupus), anemia, asthma, epilepsy, Parkinson's disease, kidney stones, or a history of heart disease or alcohol abuse. Use of naproxen may cause complications in patients with liver or kidney disease, since these organs work together to remove the medication from the body.

⇓ SIDE EFFECTS ⇓

SERIOUS
Shortness of breath or wheezing, with or without swelling of legs or other signs of heart failure; chest pain; peptic ulcer disease with vomiting of blood; black, tarry stools; decreasing kidney function. Call your doctor immediately.

COMMON
Nausea, vomiting, heartburn, diarrhea, constipation, headache, dizziness, sleepiness.

LESS COMMON
Ulcers or sores in mouth, depression, rashes or blistering of skin, ringing sound in the ears, unusual tingling or numbness of the hands or feet, seizures, blurred vision. Also elevated potassium levels, decreased blood counts; such problems can be detected by your doctor.

NEOMYCIN/POLYMYXIN B/BACITRACIN TOPICAL

Available in: Ointment
Available as Generic? Yes
Drug Class: Antibiotic combination

▼ USAGE INFORMATION

WHY IT'S TAKEN
To help prevent bacterial skin infections following minor cuts, abrasions, or burns.

HOW IT WORKS
This is a combination drug that contains three distinct antibiotics. Each of these drugs attacks and kills bacteria in a different way. Their combined, overlapping effect is capable of warding off infection by a variety of bacterial organisms.

▼ DOSAGE GUIDELINES

RANGE AND FREQUENCY
The usual treatment is to apply the ointment 2 to 5 times a day to areas of the skin that have suffered a minor injury. If you are using the prescription-strength form of the medication, follow your doctor's orders carefully; for over-the-counter forms, follow the directions.

ONSET OF EFFECT
Unknown.

DURATION OF ACTION
Unknown.

DIETARY ADVICE
This medication can be used without regard to diet.

STORAGE
Store in a tightly sealed container away from heat and direct light. Keep away from moisture and extremes in temperature.

MISSED DOSE
Apply it as soon as you remember. However, if it is near the time for the next dose, skip the missed dose and resume your regular dosage schedule. Do not apply a double dose.

STOPPING THE DRUG
Use as prescribed for the full treatment period, even if the affected area begins to look and feel better before the scheduled end of therapy. If you stop treatment prematurely, the heartier strains of bacteria are likely to survive, reproduce, and cause a worse infection later (known as a rebound infection).

PROLONGED USE
Consult your physician if you must use this medicine for a prolonged period.

▼ PRECAUTIONS

Over 60: No special precautions for older patients.

Driving and Hazardous Work: No special precautions are necessary.

Alcohol: No special precautions are necessary.

Pregnancy: Clinical studies of the use of this medication during pregnancy have not been done. Consult your doctor if you become or are planning to become pregnant.

Breast Feeding: It is not known whether this combination antibiotic passes into breast milk; caution is advised. Consult your doctor for specific advice.

Infants and Children: There is no information about use of this combination antibiotic in infants and children. However, no special problems are expected in this group.

Special Concerns: Do not use this medication if you have a history of allergic reaction to any of the active or inactive ingredients in the ointment. If you're applying this medicine without a prescription, do not use it to treat puncture wounds, deep wounds, serious burns, or raw areas unless you have first consulted your doctor. Do not use this medicine in the eyes. Before you apply the medication, wash the affected area with soap and water and dry thoroughly. You may cover the treated area with a gauze bandage if you desire.

OVERDOSE
Symptoms: No specific ones have been reported.

What to Do: While no cases of overdose have been reported, if someone accidentally ingests this medicine, call your doctor, emergency medical services (EMS), or the nearest poison control center.

▼ INTERACTIONS

DRUG INTERACTIONS
Do not use other topical medications with this preparation unless otherwise instructed by your doctor.

FOOD INTERACTIONS
No known food interactions.

DISEASE INTERACTIONS
No disease interactions have been reported with the use of this combination antibiotic.

≡ SIDE EFFECTS ≡

▼ SERIOUS
Rare, severe allergic reaction that may cause breathing difficulty or, at the extreme, total closure of the airways with potentially fatal anaphylactic shock. Contact emergency medical services (EMS) immediately. In very rare cases hearing loss may occur; if so, call your doctor immediately.

COMMON
No common side effects are associated with this medicine.

LESS COMMON
Irritation or skin allergy with burning, stinging, itching, redness, or rash. Contact your doctor as soon as possible if such side effects persist.

NICOTINE

Available in: Chewing gum, skin patch
Available as Generic? Yes
Drug Class: Smoking deterrent

▼ USAGE INFORMATION

WHY IT'S TAKEN
To reduce nicotine withdrawal symptoms as part of a comprehensive program for smoking cessation.

HOW IT WORKS
It replaces the nicotine that would otherwise be taken in by tobacco use.

▼ DOSAGE GUIDELINES

RANGE AND FREQUENCY
Used when you have the desire to smoke. Chewing gum: 20 to 24 mg a day; not to exceed 24 pieces of gum a day. Number of sticks is gradually reduced. Skin patch: To start, 1 patch supplying 22 to 24 mg a day. Dose is gradually reduced over 2 to 5 months.

ONSET OF EFFECT
30 minutes to 2 hours.

DURATION OF ACTION
3 to 6 hours.

DIETARY ADVICE
Gum should be chewed slowly over 30 minutes. Other forms can be used without regard to diet.

STORAGE
Store in a tightly sealed container away from heat and direct light.

MISSED DOSE
If you are on a specific regimen, take a missed dose as soon as you remember. If it is near the time for the next dose, skip the missed dose and resume your regular dosage schedule. Otherwise, nicotine is taken as needed.

STOPPING THE DRUG
The decision to stop taking the drug should be made in consultation with your doctor. Dose for the patch should be tapered as directed.

PROLONGED USE
Treatment should generally not exceed 2 to 6 months. If relapse of smoking occurs, treatment may be repeated.

▼ PRECAUTIONS

Over 60: Adverse reactions are not expected to be more severe in older patients than in younger persons.

Driving and Hazardous Work: The use of nicotine should not impair your ability to perform such tasks safely.

Alcohol: No special warnings.

Pregnancy: Nicotine should not be used during pregnancy. Before you use this drug, tell your doctor if you are pregnant or plan to become pregnant.

Breast Feeding: Nicotine passes into breast milk; do not use it while nursing.

Infants and Children: Should not be used. Even small amounts of nicotine can cause serious problems in infants and children.

Special Concerns: When disposing of patches or gum, be sure to use a method that keeps them out of the reach of children and animals. You should not smoke while being treated with nicotine. Do not apply a patch in the same place for at least a week.

OVERDOSE
Symptoms: Nausea, vomiting, increased salivation, severe abdominal or stomach pain, diarrhea, severe headache, cold sweats, severe dizziness, hearing and vision disturbances, confusion, weakness, breathing difficulty, heartbeat irregularities, seizures, loss of consciousness.

What to Do: Call your doctor, emergency medical services (EMS), or the nearest poison control center immediately.

▼ INTERACTIONS

DRUG INTERACTIONS
Other drugs may interact with nicotine. Consult your doctor for specific advice if you are taking aminophylline, insulin, oxtriphylline, propoxyphene, or theophylline.

FOOD INTERACTIONS
No known food interactions.

DISEASE INTERACTIONS
Caution is advised when taking nicotine. Consult your doctor if you have a history of diabetes, dental problems (with gum), heart or blood vessel disease, inflamed mouth or throat (with gum), skin allergies (with patch), an overactive thyroid, pheochromocytoma, or stomach ulcer.

☰ SIDE EFFECTS ☰

SERIOUS
With gum: Injury to mouth, dental work, or teeth. Call your dentist. With patch: Hives, itching, skin rash, or swelling. Call your doctor immediately.

COMMON
Mild headache, rapid heartbeat, increased appetite, increased salivation (with gum), sore mouth or throat, pain in jaw or neck, tooth problems (with gum and inhaler), belching (with gum), redness, burning, or itching at site of application (with patch), stinging in the nose (nasal spray).

LESS COMMON
Constipation, diarrhea, lightheadedness, dry mouth, hiccups (with gum), coughing (with inhaler), hoarseness (with gum and nasal spray), nervousness, irritability, loss of appetite, menstrual pain, joint or muscle pain, stomach upset, sweating, insomnia, unusual dreams, runny nose (with inhaler).

NIZATIDINE

BRAND NAMES

Axid, Axid AR

Available in: Capsules, tablets
Available as Generic? No
Drug Class: Histamine (H2) blocker

▼ USAGE INFORMATION

WHY IT'S TAKEN
To treat and prevent the return of ulcers of the stomach and duodenum, as well as conditions that cause increased stomach acid production (as in Zollinger-Ellison syndrome), gastroesophageal reflux (backwash of stomach acid into the esophagus, resulting in heartburn), and minor episodes of heartburn.

HOW IT WORKS
Nizatidine blocks the action of histamine (a compound produced in the body's cells), which in turn decreases the stomach's secretion of hydrochloric acid. Once stomach acid production has been decreased, the body is better able to heal itself.

▼ DOSAGE GUIDELINES

RANGE AND FREQUENCY
Adults and teenagers –To treat stomach ulcers: 300 mg once a day at bedtime, or 150 mg twice a day. To pre-vent duodenal ulcer recur-rence: 150 mg once a day at bedtime. To treat gastro-esophageal reflux: 150 mg, 2 times a day. To prevent minor cases of heartburn, acid indigestion, and sour stomach: 75 mg taken 30 to 60 minutes before a meal, once a day.

ONSET OF EFFECT
Within 30 minutes.

DURATION OF ACTION
Up to 12 hours.

DIETARY ADVICE
If you are taking two doses of nizatidine a day, the first dose can be taken after breakfast. Avoid foods that can cause stomach irritation.

STORAGE
Store in a tightly sealed con-tainer away from heat and direct light.

MISSED DOSE
Take it as soon as you remember. If it is near the time for the next dose, skip the missed dose and resume your regular dosage schedule. Do not double the next dose.

STOPPING THE DRUG
Take the prescription-strength form for the full treatment period, even if you begin to feel better before the sched-uled end of therapy.

PROLONGED USE
Do not take the maximum daily dosage continually for more than 2 weeks unless directed by your doctor.

▼ PRECAUTIONS

Over 60: Adverse reactions may be more likely and more severe in older patients.

Driving and Hazardous Work: Do not drive or engage in hazardous work until you determine how the medicine affects you.

Alcohol: Avoid alcohol.

Pregnancy: Risks vary, depending on patient and dosage. Consult your doctor.

Breast Feeding: Nizatidine passes into breast milk and may pose harm to the child; avoid or discontinue use while nursing.

Infants and Children: Nizati-dine is not recommended for young patients, although it has not been shown to cause side effects or problems dif-ferent from those in adults when used for short periods of time.

Special Concerns: Avoid cigarette smoking because it may increase stomach acid secretion and thus worsen the disease. Do not take nizatidine if you have ever had an allergic reaction to a histamine H2 blocker. If your stomach pain becomes worse while using the drug, be sure to tell your doctor right away.

OVERDOSE
Symptoms: No cases of over-dose have been reported.

What to Do: Although an overdose is unlikely, if some-one takes a much larger dose than prescribed, call your doctor, emergency medical services (EMS), or the near-est poison control center right away.

▼ INTERACTIONS

DRUG INTERACTIONS
No significant drug interac-tions have been identified. However, nizatidine may increase blood levels of aspirin. Consult your doctor for specific advice if you are taking aspirin.

FOOD INTERACTIONS
Tomato-based mixed veg-etable juices, carbonated drinks, citrus fruits and juices, caffeine-containing beverages, and other acidic foods or liq-uids may irritate the stomach or interfere with the therapeu-tic action of nizatidine.

DISEASE INTERACTIONS
Patients with kidney disease should not use nizatidine or should use it in smaller, lim-ited doses under careful supervision by a physician.

≡ SIDE EFFECTS ≡

SERIOUS
Irregular heart rhythm (palpitations), slowed heartbeat, severe blood problems, resulting in unusual bleeding, bruising, fever, chills, and increased susceptibility to infec-tion. Call your doctor immediately.

COMMON
Headache, fatigue, drowsiness, dizziness, nausea, vomiting, abdominal pain, diarrhea, constipation.

LESS COMMON
Blurred vision, decreased sexual desire or function, swelling of breasts in males and females, temporary hair loss, hallucinations, depression, insomnia, skin rash, hives, or redness.

OXYMETAZOLINE NASAL

Available in: Nasal drops, nasal spray
Available as Generic? Yes
Drug Class: Decongestant

▼ USAGE INFORMATION

WHY IT'S TAKEN
To relieve nasal congestion caused by allergies, colds, or sinus conditions.

HOW IT WORKS
Oxymetazoline constricts blood vessels to reduce the blood flow to swollen nasal passages and other upper-airway tissues, which reduces nasal secretions and improves nasal airflow.

▼ DOSAGE GUIDELINES

RANGE AND FREQUENCY
Adults and children 6 years of age and older: 2 or 3 drops or sprays of 0.05% solution in each nostril 2 times a day, in the morning and evening. Children ages 2 to 6: 2 or 3 drops of 0.025% solution in each nostril 2 times a day, in the morning and evening.

ONSET OF EFFECT
Rapid.

DURATION OF ACTION
Unknown.

DIETARY ADVICE
Drink plenty of fluids.

STORAGE
Store in a tightly sealed container away from heat and direct light.

MISSED DOSE
Take it as soon as you remember. If it is near the time for the next dose, skip the missed dose and resume your regular dosage schedule. Do not double the next dose.

STOPPING THE DRUG
Do not use this medicine for more than 3 days without consulting your doctor.

PROLONGED USE
Using this medicine for more than 3 days may lead to rebound congestion (more severe congestion caused by the body's adaptation to the drug) when you stop.

▼ PRECAUTIONS

Over 60:
Although no studies have specifically examined the use of this drug in older patients, no special problems are expected.

Driving and Hazardous Work:
Do not drive or engage in hazardous work until you determine how the medicine affects you.

Alcohol:
Avoid alcohol.

Pregnancy:
Oxymetazoline has not been shown to cause birth defects or any other problems when taken during pregnancy.

Breast Feeding:
It is not known whether oxymetazoline passes into breast milk; caution is advised. Consult your doctor for advice.

Infants and Children:
This drug is not recommended for children under the age of 2.

Special Concerns:
Each container of medicine should be used by only one person to avoid spread of infection. Blow your nose gently before using this medicine. To use the nose drops, tilt your head back or lie down on a bed and hang your head over the side. Keep your head tilted back for a few minutes after instilling the drops. To use the nasal spray, keep your head upright and sniff briskly while spraying. For best results, spray again in 3 to 5 minutes.

OVERDOSE
Symptoms: Rapid, irregular, or pounding heartbeat; headache or dizziness; increased sweating; nervousness; trembling; paleness; insomnia. Such symptoms are more likely to be seen in young children.

What to Do: If someone takes a much larger dose than recommended, call your doctor, emergency medical services (EMS), or the nearest poison control center immediately.

▼ INTERACTIONS

DRUG INTERACTIONS
Before you take oxymetazoline, tell your doctor if you are taking maprotiline or tricyclic antidepressants.

FOOD INTERACTIONS
No known food interactions.

DISEASE INTERACTIONS
Consult your doctor if you have a history of any of the following: high blood pressure, diabetes mellitus, heart disease, blood vessel disease, or an overactive thyroid gland.

≣ SIDE EFFECTS ≣

SERIOUS
No serious side effects have been reported.

COMMON
Burning, dryness, or stinging inside the nose. An increase in nasal discharge or congestion may occur after 3 to 5 days of continuous use.

LESS COMMON
Headache, rapid or irregular heartbeat, unusual excitability, restlessness.

OXYMETAZOLINE OPHTHALMIC

OcuClear, Visine L.R.

Available in: Ophthalmic solution
Available as Generic? No
Drug Class: Ophthalmic decongestant

▼ USAGE INFORMATION

WHY IT'S TAKEN
To reduce redness of the eye caused by minor irritation.

HOW IT WORKS
Ophthalmic oxymetazoline reduces redness by constricting the superficial blood vessels in the whites (sclera) of the eye.

▼ DOSAGE GUIDELINES

RANGE AND FREQUENCY
Adults and children age 6 and older: 1 drop in the affected eye every 6 hours, as needed.

ONSET OF EFFECT
Rapid, within 5 minutes.

DURATION OF ACTION
About 6 hours.

DIETARY ADVICE
No special restrictions.

STORAGE
Store in a tightly sealed container away from moisture, heat, and direct light. Do not allow the medicine to freeze.

MISSED DOSE
Apply it as soon as you remember. However, if it is near the time for the next dose, skip the missed dose and resume your regular dosage schedule. Do not double the next dose.

STOPPING THE DRUG
Do not use this medicine for more than 3 days without consulting your doctor.

PROLONGED USE
Consult your doctor if you intend to use this medicine for more than 3 days.

▼ PRECAUTIONS

Over 60: Although no studies have specifically examined the use of this drug in older patients, no special problems are expected.

Driving and Hazardous Work: Do not drive or engage in hazardous work until you determine how the medicine affects you.

Alcohol: No special warnings.

Pregnancy: No problems are expected, but studies of effects in pregnancy have not been done in humans. Consult your physician.

Breast Feeding: No problems are expected, but studies of effects in breast feeding have not been done in humans. Consult your doctor.

Infants and Children: Dosage for children under the age of 6 should be determined by a pediatrician.

Special Concerns: To use the eye drops, first wash your hands. Tilt your head back. Gently apply pressure to the inside corner of the eyelid and with the index finger of the same hand, pull downward on the lower eyelid to make a space. Drop the medicine into this space and close your eye. Apply pressure for 1 or 2 minutes while keeping the eye closed without blinking. Then wash your hands again. To avoid contamination, be sure the tip of the dropper does not touch your eye, finger, or any other surface.

OVERDOSE
Symptoms: Dizziness; headache; rapid, irregular, or pounding heartbeat; trembling; insomnia.

What to Do: Call your doctor, emergency medical services (EMS), or the nearest poison control center immediately.

▼ INTERACTIONS

DRUG INTERACTIONS
Before you take oxymetazoline, tell your doctor if you are taking maprotiline or tricyclic antidepressants.

FOOD INTERACTIONS
No known food interactions.

DISEASE INTERACTIONS
Caution is advised when taking oxymetazoline. Consult your doctor if you have a history of any of the following: high blood pressure; eye disease, infection, or injury; narrow-angle glaucoma; heart disease; blood vessel disease; or an overactive thyroid gland.

≡ SIDE EFFECTS ≡

▼ SERIOUS ▼
No serious side effects have been reported.

COMMON
No common side effects have been reported.

LESS COMMON
Headache, rapid or irregular heartbeat, excitability, restlessness, increase in redness of the eye.

PERMETHRIN

BRAND NAMES

Elimite, Nix

Available in: Lotion
Available as Generic? Yes
Drug Class: Topical antiparasitic

▼ USAGE INFORMATION

WHY IT'S TAKEN
To treat head lice infestations.

HOW IT WORKS
Permethrin is absorbed into the bodies of lice, where it blocks nerve activity, ultimately causing paralysis and death of the lice. (The drug does not have this toxic effect on humans.)

▼ DOSAGE GUIDELINES

RANGE AND FREQUENCY
For treatment of head lice (pediculus humanus capitus): After the hair has been washed with shampoo, rinsed with water, and dried with a towel, apply a sufficient amount (approximately 25 ml) of liquid. Allow it to remain on the hair for 10 minutes, then rinse off with water. Rinse thoroughly and dry with a clean towel. Use a fine-tooth comb to remove any remaining nits or nit shells. If lice are found after 7 days, repeat the treatment.

ONSET OF EFFECT
Within 10 minutes.

DURATION OF ACTION
Up to 10 days.

DIETARY ADVICE
Permethrin can be used without regard to diet.

STORAGE
Store in a tightly sealed container away from heat and direct light.

MISSED DOSE
If a second dose is needed and you do not administer it after 7 days, do so as soon as you remember.

STOPPING THE DRUG
You need not take the second dose if no lice are found after 7 days.

PROLONGED USE
If lice recur, consult your doctor.

▼ PRECAUTIONS

Over 60: No special problems are expected.

Driving and Hazardous Work: The use of permethrin should not impair your ability to perform such tasks safely.

Alcohol: No special warnings.

Pregnancy: In animal studies, permethrin has not caused problems or birth defects. Human studies have not been done. Before you use permethrin, tell your doctor if you are pregnant or plan to become pregnant.

Breast Feeding: Permethrin may pass into breast milk; caution is advised. Consult your doctor for advice.

Infants and Children: Use and dosage in children up to 2 years of age must be determined by your doctor.

Special Concerns: All members of your household should be examined for lice and given treatment if necessary. Any sexual partner should be examined and treated if necessary. Clothing, household linen, hairbrushes, combs, and bedding should be thoroughly cleaned by machine washing with hot water and machine drying for at least 20 minutes, using the hot cycle. Seal nonwashable items in a plastic bag for at least 2 weeks or spray them with a product designed to eliminate lice and their nits. You should not use this drug if you are hypersensitive to chrysanthemums. Treatment with permethrin may temporarily worsen the itching and other symptoms of head lice infestation.

OVERDOSE
Symptoms: No cases of overdose have been reported.

What to Do: Although overdose is unlikely, if someone accidentally ingests the drug, call your doctor, emergency medical services (EMS), or the nearest poison control center immediately.

▼ INTERACTIONS

DRUG INTERACTIONS
Before you use this medicine, tell your doctor if you are using any other prescription or over-the-counter medication that is to be applied to the scalp.

FOOD INTERACTIONS
No known food interactions.

DISEASE INTERACTIONS
Consult your doctor if you have severe inflammation of the skin.

≡ SIDE EFFECTS ≡

SERIOUS
No serious side effects have been reported.

COMMON
Burning, itching, numbness, rash, redness, stinging, swelling, or tingling of scalp. In most cases such symptoms are mild and temporary; notify your doctor if they are more troublesome or if they persist.

LESS COMMON
No less-common side effects have been reported.

PHENAZOPYRIDINE HYDROCHLORIDE

Azo-Standard, Baridium, Eridium, Geridium, Phenazodine, Pyridiate, Pyridium, Urodine, Urogesic, Viridium

Available in: Tablets
Available as Generic? Yes
Drug Class: Urinary analgesic

▼ USAGE INFORMATION

WHY IT'S TAKEN
For short-term relief of symptoms caused by irritation of the urinary tract. Such symptoms include burning, pain, and discomfort during urination, as well as an increased urge to urinate with only small amounts of urine passed on each occasion. Irritation of the urinary tract commonly occurs as a result of bladder infection; phenazopyridine can ease symptoms but will not cure such an infection.

HOW IT WORKS
Phenazopyridine passes through—and has a local anesthetic effect upon the lining of—the urinary tract, thus relieving the discomfort associated with urinary infection or inflammation.

▼ DOSAGE GUIDELINES

RANGE AND FREQUENCY
Adults: 200 mg, 3 times a day. Children: 1.8 mg per lb of body weight, 3 times a day.

ONSET OF EFFECT
Unknown.

DURATION OF ACTION
Unknown.

DIETARY ADVICE
This medication is best taken with or after meals to minimize stomach upset.

STORAGE
Store in a tightly sealed container away from moisture, heat, and direct light.

MISSED DOSE
Take it as soon as you remember. If it is near the time for the next dose, skip the missed dose and resume your regular dosage schedule. Do not double the next dose.

STOPPING THE DRUG
The decision to stop taking the drug should be made by your doctor. If it is being taken with an antibiotic, it should be taken for only 2 days (6 doses).

PROLONGED USE
Phenazopyridine is intended only for short-term use.

▼ PRECAUTIONS

Over 60: No special problems are expected.

Driving and Hazardous Work: Do not drive or engage in hazardous work until you determine how the medicine affects you.

Alcohol: No special precautions are necessary.

Pregnancy: Adequate human studies have not been done. Before taking phenazopyridine, tell your doctor if you are pregnant or plan to become pregnant.

Breast Feeding: Phenazopyridine may pass into breast milk; caution is advised. Consult your doctor for advice.

Infants and Children: No special problems are expected.

Special Concerns: Phenazopyridine causes the urine to turn reddish orange. This is harmless, but it may stain clothing. The drug may also cause permanent staining or discoloration of soft contact lenses; it is best to wear glasses while taking the drug. For diabetic patients, phenazopyridine may cause false test results with sugar and urine ketone tests. Do not chew the tablets; chewing may cause permanent discoloration of teeth. Do not use any leftover medicine for future urinary tract infections without consulting your doctor.

OVERDOSE
Symptoms: Fatigue, paleness, shortness of breath, heart palpitations, bloody or cloudy urine, decreased urine output, swelling of the ankles and calves, lower back or flank pain, nausea or vomiting.

What to Do: While an overdose is unlikely, call your doctor, emergency medical services (EMS), or the nearest poison control center immediately if any symptoms of overdose occur.

▼ INTERACTIONS

DRUG INTERACTIONS
Some drugs may interact with phenazopyridine. Consult your doctor for specific advice if you are taking any prescription or over-the-counter medication.

FOOD INTERACTIONS
No known food interactions.

DISEASE INTERACTIONS
Caution is advised when taking phenazopyridine. Consult your doctor if you have any of the following: hepatitis, glucose-6-phosphate dehydrogenase deficiency (G6PD) uremia, pyelonephritis (kidney infection) during pregnancy, or other kidney disease.

⎯ SIDE EFFECTS ⎯

SERIOUS
Serious side effects are rare. Call your doctor immediately if you experience any of the following: difficulty breathing, swelling of the face, fingers, feet, or lower legs, blue or purple-blue skin color, unusual fatigue, fever, confusion, sudden decrease in urine output, shortness of breath, tightness in the chest, skin rash, yellow discoloration of the eyes or skin, unusual weight gain.

COMMON
Reddish orange urine.

LESS COMMON
Indigestion, dizziness, stomach cramps or pain, headache.

PHENYLEPHRINE HYDROCHLORIDE OPHTHALMIC

Available in: Ophthalmic solution
Available as Generic? Yes
Drug Class: Adrenergic agent

▼ USAGE INFORMATION

WHY IT'S TAKEN
The 2.5% and 10% solutions are used to dilate the pupil of the eye (prior to eye examinations or ophthalmologic procedures) and to treat certain eye conditions. The 0.12 % solution is recommended to reduce redness of the eye that is caused by minor irritation.

HOW IT WORKS
Ophthalmic phenylephrine affects the muscles that control the pupils. causing them to dilate, which helps the doctor view the interior structures of the eye. The drug reduces redness by constricting the superficial blood vessels in the whites of the eye.

▼ DOSAGE GUIDELINES

RANGE AND FREQUENCY
For redness—Adults and children: 1 drop of 0.12% solution every 3 or 4 hours as needed.

ONSET OF EFFECT
Rapid.

DURATION OF ACTION
From 2 to 7 hours depending on the strength of the solution used.

DIETARY ADVICE
No special precautions.

STORAGE
Store in a tightly sealed container away from moisture, heat, and direct light. Do not allow the medicine to freeze.

MISSED DOSE
Apply it as soon as you remember. If it is near the time for the next dose, skip the missed dose and resume your regular dosage schedule. Do not double the next dose.

STOPPING THE DRUG
The decision to stop using the drug should be made by your doctor.

PROLONGED USE
You should see your doctor regularly if you must use this drug for an extended period of time.

▼ PRECAUTIONS

Over 60: No special advice.

Driving and Hazardous Work: Do not drive or engage in hazardous work until you determine how the medicine affects your vision.

Alcohol: No special precautions are necessary.

Pregnancy: No problems are expected, but studies of effects in pregnancy have not been done in humans. Consult your physician.

Breast Feeding: No problems are expected, but studies of effects in breast feeding have not been done in humans. Consult your doctor.

Infants and Children: Adverse reactions may be more likely and more severe in infants and children. The 10% solution should not be used on infants. The other strengths should not be used on low-birth-weight infants.

Special Concerns: To use the eye drops, first wash your hands. Tilt your head back. Gently apply pressure to the inside corner of the eyelid and with the index finger of the same hand, pull downward on the lower eyelid to make a space. Drop the medicine into this space and close your eye. Apply pressure for 1 or 2 minutes while keeping the eye closed without blinking. Then wash your hands again. Make sure the tip of the dropper does not touch your eye, finger, or any other surface. Phenylephrine will make your eyes more sensitive to sunlight. If this occurs, wear sunglasses or avoid bright light as comfort dictates. If this effect continues for more than 12 hours after you have stopped the medicine, consult your doctor.

▼ OVERDOSE

Symptoms: Dizziness; paleness; rapid, irregular, or pounding heartbeat; trembling; profuse sweating; vomiting; coma; shock.

What to Do: Call your doctor, emergency medical services (EMS), or the nearest poison control center immediately.

▼ INTERACTIONS

DRUG INTERACTIONS
Be sure to tell your doctor if you are using any other prescription or OTC medication.

FOOD INTERACTIONS
No known food interactions.

DISEASE INTERACTIONS
Consult your doctor if you have a history of heart disease, blood vessel disease, diabetes mellitus, high blood pressure, or idiopathic orthostatic hypotension (low blood pressure). This drug should not be used by those with a history of closed-angle glaucoma.

☰ SIDE EFFECTS ☰

SERIOUS
Dizziness; paleness; rapid, irregular, or pounding heartbeat; trembling; increased sweating. Call your doctor immediately.

COMMON
Unusually large pupils; burning, stinging, or watering of eyes; sensitivity of eyes to light; headache or brow ache.

LESS COMMON
Eye irritation not present prior to therapy.

PHENYLEPHRINE HYDROCHLORIDE SYSTEMIC

Available in: Nasal jelly, nasal drops, nasal spray
Available as Generic? Yes
Drug Class: Decongestant

▼ USAGE INFORMATION

WHY IT'S TAKEN
To relieve nasal congestion caused by allergies, colds, or sinus conditions; to relieve congestion associated with ear infections.

HOW IT WORKS
Phenylephrine constricts blood vessels to reduce blood flow to swollen nasal passages, which reduces nasal secretions and improves airflow.

▼ DOSAGE GUIDELINES

RANGE AND FREQUENCY
Adults and children 12 and over: 2 to 3 drops of 0.25% to 0.5% solution, or 1 to 2 sprays, or a small amount of jelly in each nostril every 4 hours. Children 6 to 12 years: 2 to 3 drops or 1 to 2 sprays of a 0.25% solution in each nostril every 4 hours. Children under 6 years: 2 to 3 drops of 0.125% solution every 4 hours.

ONSET OF EFFECT
Rapid.

DURATION OF ACTION
From 30 minutes to 4 hours.

DIETARY ADVICE
Drink plenty of fluids.

STORAGE
Store in a tightly sealed container away from heat and direct light.

MISSED DOSE
Take it as soon as you remember. If it is near the time for the next dose, skip the missed dose and resume your regular dosage schedule. Do not double the next dose.

STOPPING THE DRUG
Do not take this medicine for more than 3 days without consulting your doctor about its use.

PROLONGED USE
Using this medicine for more than 3 days may lead to rebound congestion (more severe congestion caused by the body's adaptation to the drug).

▼ PRECAUTIONS

Over 60: Although no studies have specifically examined the use of this drug in older patients, no special problems are expected.

Driving and Hazardous Work: Do not drive or engage in hazardous work until you determine how the medicine affects you.

Alcohol: Avoid alcohol.

Pregnancy: Phenylephrine hydrochloride has not been shown to cause birth defects or other problems if taken during pregnancy.

Breast Feeding: It is not known whether phenylephrine passes into breast milk; caution is advised. Consult your doctor for advice.

Infants and Children: Adverse reactions may be more likely and more severe in infants and children.

Special Concerns: Each container of medicine should be used by only one person to avoid spread of infection. Blow your nose gently before using this medicine. To use the nose drops, tilt your head back or lie down on a bed and hang your head over the side. Keep your head tilted back for a few minutes after instilling the drops. To use the nasal spray, keep your head upright and sniff briskly while spraying. For best results, spray again in 3 to 5 minutes. To use the nasal jelly, first wash your hands, then place an amount of jelly about the size of a pea into each nostril and sniff it well back into the nose.

OVERDOSE
Symptoms: Rapid, irregular, or pounding heartbeat; headache or dizziness; increased sweating; nervousness; trembling; paleness; insomnia. Such symptoms are more likely to be seen in young children.

What to Do: If someone takes a much larger dose than recommended, call your doctor, emergency medical services (EMS), or the nearest poison control center immediately.

▼ INTERACTIONS

DRUG INTERACTIONS
Before you take phenylephrine, tell your doctor if you are taking any other prescription or OTC drug.

FOOD INTERACTIONS
No known food interactions.

DISEASE INTERACTIONS
Consult your doctor if you have a history of any of the following: high blood pressure, diabetes mellitus, heart disease, blood vessel (vascular) disease, or an overactive thyroid gland.

≣ SIDE EFFECTS ≣

SERIOUS
No serious side effects have been reported.

COMMON
Burning, dryness, or stinging inside the nose. An increase in nasal discharge or congestion may occur after 3 to 5 days of continuous use.

LESS COMMON
Headache, rapid or irregular heartbeat, excitability, restlessness.

PSEUDOEPHEDRINE

Available in: Extended-release capsules, oral solution, syrup, tablets
Available as Generic? Yes
Drug Class: Decongestant/cough drug

▼ USAGE INFORMATION

WHY IT'S TAKEN
To relieve nasal or sinus congestion caused by colds, sinus infection, hay fever, or other respiratory allergies.

HOW IT WORKS
Pseudoephedrine narrows and constricts blood vessels to reduce the blood flow to swollen nasal passages and other tissues, which reduces nasal secretions, shrinks swollen nasal mucous membranes, and improves airflow in nasal passages.

▼ DOSAGE GUIDELINES

RANGE AND FREQUENCY
Short-acting forms—Adults and teenagers: 60 mg every 4 to 6 hours; not more than 240 mg in 24 hours. Children 6 to 12 years of age: 30 mg every 4 to 6 hours; not more than 120 mg in 24 hours. Children 2 to 6 years of age: 15 mg every 4 hours; not more than 60 mg in 24 hours. Extended-release form—Adults and teenagers: 120 mg every 12 hours or 240 mg every 24 hours.

ONSET OF EFFECT
15 to 30 minutes.

DURATION OF ACTION
3 to 4 hours for short-acting forms, 8 to 12 hours for extended-release form.

DIETARY ADVICE
Drink plenty of fluids.

STORAGE
Store in a tightly sealed container away from heat and direct light. Do not allow the liquid form to freeze.

MISSED DOSE
Take it as soon as you remember. If it is near the time for the next dose, skip the missed dose and resume your regular dosage schedule. Do not double the next dose.

STOPPING THE DRUG
Do not take this drug longer than recommended on the label unless directed to do so by your doctor.

PROLONGED USE
Consult your doctor about taking pseudoephedrine for more than 5 to 7 days.

▼ PRECAUTIONS

Over 60: Side effects may be more likely and more severe in elderly patients.

Driving and Hazardous Work: Avoid such activities until you determine how the medicine affects you.

Alcohol: No special precautions are necessary.

Pregnancy: Safety has not been established; it should be used only if clearly necessary. Consult your doctor for specific advice.

Breast Feeding: Pseudoephedrine passes into breast milk; avoid or discontinue use while nursing.

Infants and Children: Use of extended-release forms of pseudoephedrine is not recommended for children under the age of 12.

Special Concerns: If your symptoms do not improve within 7 days, check with your doctor. To help prevent insomnia, take the last dose of the day at least 2 hours before your bedtime.

OVERDOSE
Symptoms: Drowsiness, sedation, profuse sweating, pale or clammy skin, low blood pressure, diminished urine output, dizziness, changes in mental state, hallucinations, seizures, loss of consciousness.

What to Do: In some cases an overdose can be fatal, especially among elderly patients. At the first sign of overdose, call your doctor, emergency medical services (EMS), or the nearest poison control center immediately.

▼ INTERACTIONS

DRUG INTERACTIONS
Consult your doctor for specific advice before using pseudoephedrine if you are taking beta-blockers or MAO inhibitors.

FOOD INTERACTIONS
No known food interactions.

DISEASE INTERACTIONS
Caution is advised when taking pseudoephedrine. Consult your doctor if you have any of the following: diabetes, enlarged prostate, heart disease, blood vessel disease, high blood pressure, or an overactive thyroid gland.

≣ SIDE EFFECTS ≣
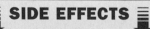

SERIOUS
Seizures, irregular or slowed heartbeat, shortness of breath, breathing difficulty, hallucinations. Stop taking the medication and call your doctor right away.

COMMON
Nervousness, restlessness, insomnia.

LESS COMMON
Difficult or painful urination, dizziness or lightheadedness, rapid or pounding heartbeat, increased sweating, nausea or vomiting, trembling, trouble breathing, paleness, weakness.

PSEUDOEPHEDRINE/GUAIFENESIN

BRAND NAMES
Deconsal II,
Deconsal LA, Entex PSE

Available in: Capsules, oral solution, syrup, tablets, extended-release forms
Available as Generic? No
Drug Class: Decongestant/cough drug

▼ USAGE INFORMATION

WHY IT'S TAKEN
To relieve nasal or sinus congestion caused by colds, influenza (flu), hay fever, and other respiratory allergies. Also intended to break up congestion in the lungs to promote better breathing.

HOW IT WORKS
Pseudoephedrine narrows and constricts blood vessels to reduce the blood flow to swollen nasal passages and other tissues, which reduces nasal secretions, shrinks swollen nasal mucous membranes, and improves airflow. Guaifenesin purportedly breaks up, liquefies, and loosens mucus secretions in the respiratory tract, making it easier to cough up phlegm and thus breathe easier. (There is some debate, however, as to whether the medication is actually effective in this regard.)

▼ DOSAGE GUIDELINES

RANGE AND FREQUENCY
Take the drug as directed to relieve symptoms.

ONSET OF EFFECT
Within 1 hour.

DURATION OF ACTION
Unknown.

DIETARY ADVICE
No special restrictions.

STORAGE
Store in a tightly sealed container away from heat and direct light.

MISSED DOSE
Take it as soon as you remember. If it is near the time for the next dose, skip the missed dose and resume your regular dosage schedule. Do not double the next dose.

STOPPING THE DRUG
The decision to stop taking the drug should be made by your doctor or when you note improvement.

PROLONGED USE
Check with your doctor if symptoms do not improve within 5 days.

▼ PRECAUTIONS

Over 60: Adverse reactions may be more likely and more severe in older patients.

Driving and Hazardous Work: Do not drive or engage in hazardous work until you determine how the medicine affects you.

Alcohol: Avoid alcohol.

Pregnancy: Before taking pseudoephedrine and guaifenesin, tell your doctor if you are pregnant or plan to become pregnant.

Breast Feeding: Pseudoephedrine passes into breast milk; avoid or discontinue use while nursing.

Infants and Children: Check the package label or with your doctor before giving it to infants or children.

Special Concerns: If you have trouble sleeping, take the last dose of pseudoephedrine and guaifenesin a few hours before bedtime. Before having any surgery, tell your doctor or dentist that you are taking this drug. Be sure your doctor knows if you have high blood pressure.

OVERDOSE
Symptoms: Rapid, pounding, or irregular heartbeat, continuing and severe headache, severe nausea or vomiting, severe nervousness or restlessness, severe shortness of breath or troubled breathing.

What to Do: Call your doctor, emergency medical services (EMS), or the nearest poison control center immediately.

▼ INTERACTIONS

DRUG INTERACTIONS
Consult your doctor if you are taking any prescription or nonprescription medication. Do not take any drug for diet or appetite control unless you have checked with your doctor first.

FOOD INTERACTIONS
No known food interactions.

DISEASE INTERACTIONS
Caution is advised when taking pseudoephedrine and guaifenesin. Consult your doctor if you have any of the following: anemia, gout, hemophilia, stomach problems, brain disease, colitis, seizures, diarrhea, gallbladder disease or gallstones, cystic fibrosis, diabetes mellitus, any chronic lung disease, enlarged prostate, difficult urination, glaucoma, heart or blood vessel disease, thyroid disease, or high blood pressure. Use of pseudoephedrine and guaifenesin may cause complications in persons with liver or kidney disease, since these organs work together to remove the medication from the body.

▦ SIDE EFFECTS ▦

SERIOUS
Skin rash, hives, itching, rapid or irregular heartbeat, persistent head-ache, nervousness or restlessness, shortness of breath or breathing difficulty, seizures, unusual fear and anxiety. Call your doctor or emergency medical services (EMS) right away.

COMMON
Constipation; decreased sweating; difficult urination; dizziness or lightheadedness; drowsiness; dry mouth, nose, or throat; increased sensitivity of skin to sun; thickened mucus; nausea or vomiting; nightmares; stomach pain; insomnia; unusual excitement or restlessness; unusual tiredness or weakness. Contact your doctor if these symptoms persist or interfere with your daily activities.

LESS COMMON
There are no less-common side effects associated with the use of this drug.

PSYLLIUM

Available in: Caramels, granules, powder
Available as Generic? Yes
Drug Class: Bulk-forming laxative

▼ USAGE INFORMATION

WHY IT'S TAKEN
To relieve constipation. It also may be prescribed for treatment of diarrhea.

HOW IT WORKS
Psyllium is a natural soluble fiber derived from the husks of a seed grain. It absorbs liquid in the intestines and swells to form a soft, bulky stool. The increased bulk of the stool stimulates bowel activity and triggers the urge to defecate. Psyllium has also been shown in studies to improve the ratio of HDL ("good") cholesterol to LDL ("bad") cholesterol in the blood. For this reason, it is sometimes prescribed as part of a program to reduce high cholesterol levels before resorting to drug therapy.

▼ DOSAGE GUIDELINES

RANGE AND FREQUENCY
Adults: 1 to 2 rounded teaspoons or 1 packet dissolved in water, 1, 2, or 3 times a day, followed by a second glass of liquid. Children over 6: 1 level teaspoon in half a glass of water.

▤ SIDE EFFECTS ▤

SERIOUS
Difficulty breathing, intestinal blockage (resulting in severe, painful constipation), skin rash or itching, difficulty swallowing. Call your doctor immediately.

COMMON
No common side effects have been reported.

LESS COMMON
Nausea, vomiting, partial intestinal obstruction, abdominal pain or cramping.

ONSET OF EFFECT
Usually, 12 to 24 hours. In some cases, up to 3 days.

DURATION OF ACTION
Variable.

DIETARY ADVICE
Take psyllium with a full glass of cold liquid, such as fruit juice or water, and follow with another full glass.

STORAGE
Store in a tightly sealed container away from moisture, heat, and direct light.

MISSED DOSE
Take it as soon as you remember. If it is near the time for the next dose, skip the missed dose and resume your regular dosage schedule. Do not double the next dose.

STOPPING THE DRUG
Take it as directed for the full treatment period. However, you may stop taking it if you are feeling better before the scheduled end of therapy.

PROLONGED USE
Do not take psyllium for more than 1 week unless your doctor has ordered a special schedule for you.

▼ PRECAUTIONS

Over 60: No special advice.

Driving and Hazardous Work: No special warnings.

Alcohol: Avoid alcohol; it can irritate the gastrointestinal tract and interfere with proper digestion.

Pregnancy: Discuss with your doctor the relative risks and benefits of using psyllium while pregnant.

Breast Feeding: Psyllium may pass into breast milk; caution is advised. Consult your doctor for advice.

Infants and Children: Not recommended for use by children under age 6.

Special Concerns: You should have an adequate amount of fiber-containing food in your diet, such as cereals, fresh fruit, and vegetables. Before you take psyllium, tell your doctor if you have had any unusual or allergic reaction to laxatives. Make sure that your doctor knows if you are on any special diet. Do not take any other medicine within 2 hours of taking psyllium. Drink from 6 to 8 eight-ounce glasses of water every day.

OVERDOSE
Symptoms: Intestinal blockage if psyllium is taken in excessive doses.

What to Do: An overdose of psyllium is unlikely. However, if someone takes a much larger dose than prescribed, seek medical help promptly.

▼ INTERACTIONS

DRUG INTERACTIONS
Consult your doctor for advice if you are taking oral tetracyclines.

FOOD INTERACTIONS
Psyllium may interfere with the absorption of certain minerals, especially in high doses or with regular use.

DISEASE INTERACTIONS
Consult your doctor before using psyllium if you have any of the following: heart disease, a colostomy or ileostomy, diabetes mellitus, high blood pressure, kidney disease, rectal bleeding of unknown cause, difficulty swallowing, or any signs of appendicitis.

PYRANTEL PAMOATE

Available in: Oral suspension
Available as Generic? Yes
Drug Class: Anthelmintic

▼ USAGE INFORMATION

WHY IT'S TAKEN
To treat various worm infections, including ascariasis (common roundworm) and enterobiasis or oxyuriasis (pinworm). It may be used to treat more than one worm infection at a time. It may also be used for other types of infection as determined by your doctor.

HOW IT WORKS
Pyrantel paralyzes the worm. While it is paralyzed, the worm is expelled from the body in the stool.

▼ DOSAGE GUIDELINES

RANGE AND FREQUENCY
Adults and children age 2 and older—For roundworms: 1 dose of 11 mg per 2.2 lbs (1 kg) of body weight. Maximum dose is 1,000 mg. If necessary, the dose may be repeated in 2 to 3 weeks. For pinworms: 1 dose of 11 mg per 2.2 lbs of body weight. Maximum dose is 1,000 mg. Repeat the dose in 2 to 3 weeks.

ONSET OF EFFECT
Variable.

DURATION OF ACTION
Variable.

DIETARY ADVICE
Pyrantel can be taken with fruit juice, milk, or food.

STORAGE
Store in a tightly sealed container away from moisture, heat, and direct light. Do not allow it to freeze.

MISSED DOSE
Take a missed dose as soon as you remember.

STOPPING THE DRUG
The decision to stop taking the drug should be made in consultation with your doctor.

PROLONGED USE
Pyrantel is generally recommended for one-time use (two-time use for pinworms).

▼ PRECAUTIONS

Over 60: Adverse reactions may be more likely and more severe in older patients.

Driving and Hazardous Work: Do not drive or engage in hazardous work until you determine how the medicine affects you.

Alcohol: No special precautions are necessary.

Pregnancy: Pyrantel is not recommended for use in pregnant women. Consult your doctor for specific advice if you are pregnant or plan to become pregnant.

Breast Feeding: Pyrantel may pass into breast milk; caution is advised. Consult your doctor for advice.

Infants and Children: Use and dosage for children under the age of 2 should be determined by your doctor. Not recommended for use by children under the age of 1.

Special Concerns: To prevent reinfection, wash clothing, bedding, and towels every day. All members of the family may have to be treated to eradicate the infestation. A second treatment for all household members may be necessary after 2 or 3 weeks. All bedding and nightclothes should be washed again after treatment. To prevent reinfection, you should wash the anal region daily, change your underwear and bedding every day, and wash your hands and fingernails before each meal and after bowel movements. Consult your doctor if your condition has not improved upon completion of therapy.

OVERDOSE
Symptoms: An overdose with pyrantel is unlikely.

What to Do: If someone takes a much larger dose than directed, call your doctor, emergency medical services (EMS), or the nearest poison control center right away.

▼ INTERACTIONS

DRUG INTERACTIONS
Do not take piperazine when taking pyrantel. The effectiveness of both drugs may be reduced. Consult your doctor for specific advice. Also tell your doctor if you are taking any other prescription or OTC medication.

FOOD INTERACTIONS
No known food interactions.

DISEASE INTERACTIONS
Caution is advised when taking pyrantel. Consult your doctor for specific advice if you have any other medical condition.

≡ SIDE EFFECTS ≡

SERIOUS
Skin rash. Stop using the drug and call your doctor as soon as possible.

COMMON
No common side effects are associated with the use of pyrantel.

LESS COMMON
Pain or cramps in abdomen or stomach, headache, dizziness, diarrhea, drowsiness, insomnia, nausea or vomiting, loss of appetite.

PYRETHRINS/PIPERONYL BUTOXIDE

Available in: Gel, solution shampoo, topical solution
Available as Generic? Yes
Drug Class: Topical antiparasitic

▼ USAGE INFORMATION

WHY IT'S TAKEN
To treat head, body, and pubic lice infestations. Although this drug is available without a prescription, your doctor may have special instructions regarding its proper use.

HOW IT WORKS
Pyrethrins and piperonyl butoxide are a combination of active ingredients. The medication is absorbed into the bodies of lice, where it blocks nerve activity, ultimately causing paralysis and death of the lice. (The drug has no such toxic effect on humans.)

▼ DOSAGE GUIDELINES

RANGE AND FREQUENCY
Use 1 time, then repeat one more time in 7 to 10 days. Gel or solution: Apply enough medicine to thoroughly wet hair, scalp, or skin. Allow the medicine to remain on the affected areas for 10 minutes, then wash with warm water and soap or regular shampoo. Rinse thoroughly and dry with a clean towel. Shampoo: Apply enough medicine to wet the hair, scalp, or skin. Allow the medicine to remain on the affected areas for 10 minutes, then use a small amount of water to work shampoo more thoroughly into affected area. Rinse and dry with a clean towel. With either method, use a nit-removal comb to remove dead lice and eggs from hair.

ONSET OF EFFECT
Within 10 minutes.

DURATION OF ACTION
Up to 10 days.

DIETARY ADVICE
This medication can be used without regard to diet.

STORAGE
Store in a tightly sealed container away from heat and direct light, and away from children.

MISSED DOSE
If you do not administer the second dose within 10 days after the initial dose, do so as soon as you remember.

STOPPING THE DRUG
Take both recommended doses, even if you are feeling better before the scheduled end of therapy.

PROLONGED USE
If lice recur, consult your doctor.

▼ PRECAUTIONS

Over 60: No special problems are expected to occur in older patients.

Driving and Hazardous Work: The use of pyrethrins and piperonyl butoxide should not impair your ability to perform such tasks safely.

Alcohol: No special precautions are necessary.

Pregnancy: This drug has not been shown to cause birth defects or other problems during pregnancy. Before you use pyrethrins and piperonyl butoxide, tell your doctor if you are pregnant or plan to become pregnant.

Breast Feeding: Pyrethrins and piperonyl butoxide may pass into breast milk; caution is advised. Consult your doctor for specific information.

Infants and Children: No special problems are expected in younger patients.

Special Concerns: All members of your household should be examined for lice and given treatment if necessary. Clothing, household linen, hairbrushes, combs, and bedding should be thoroughly cleaned. Furniture, rugs, and floors should be vacuumed thoroughly. Toilet seats should be scrubbed often. If you use this medicine for pubic lice, your sexual partner may also need to be treated. Keep this medicine away from the mouth and do not inhale it. Apply it in a well-ventilated room to help prevent inhalation. Keep the medicine away from the eyes and other mucous membranes, such as the inside of the nose or vagina.

OVERDOSE
Symptoms: If accidentally ingested, pyrethrins and piperonyl butoxide can cause nausea, vomiting, muscle paralysis, and central nervous system depression.

What to Do: Call your doctor, emergency medical services (EMS), or the nearest poison control center immediately.

▼ INTERACTIONS

DRUG INTERACTIONS
Before you use this medicine, tell your doctor if you are using any other prescription or over-the-counter drugs.

FOOD INTERACTIONS
No known food interactions.

DISEASE INTERACTIONS
Consult your doctor if you have any severe inflammation of the skin.

≡ SIDE EFFECTS ≡

SERIOUS
Skin irritation not present before use of the medicine, skin rash or infection, sudden attacks of sneezing, stuffy or runny nose, wheezing or difficulty breathing. Call your doctor immediately.

COMMON
No common side effects are associated with pyrethrins and piperonyl butoxide.

LESS COMMON
No less-common side effects are associated with pyrethrins and piperonyl butoxide.

RANITIDINE

Available in: Capsules, tablets, syrup, granules
Available as Generic? Yes
Drug Class: Histamine (H2) blocker

▼ USAGE INFORMATION

WHY IT'S TAKEN
To treat ulcers of the stomach and duodenum, conditions that cause increased stomach acid production (such as Zollinger-Ellison syndrome), erosive esophagitis (severe, chronic inflammation of the esophagus), and gastro-esophageal reflux (backwash of stomach acid into the esophagus, causing heartburn).

HOW IT WORKS
Ranitidine blocks the action of histamine (a compound produced in the body's cells), which in turn decreases the stomach's secretion of hydrochloric acid. Once stomach acid production is decreased, the body is better able to heal itself.

▼ DOSAGE GUIDELINES

RANGE AND FREQUENCY
Adults—150 mg, 2 times a day, in the morning and at bedtime, or 300 mg once daily before bedtime.

Patients with Zollinger-Ellison syndrome may require up to 6 g per day (and the medication should be taken orally). For treatment of heartburn with the OTC form: 75 mg, as needed, not to exceed 150 mg a day. Children—Consult your pediatrician for the appropriate dosage for your particular child.

ONSET OF EFFECT
30 to 60 minutes.

DURATION OF ACTION
Up to 13 hours.

DIETARY ADVICE
Avoid foods that cause stomach irritation.

STORAGE
Store away from heat and direct light. Keep liquid form from freezing.

MISSED DOSE
Take it as soon as you remember. If it is near the time for the next dose, skip the missed dose and resume your regular dosage schedule. Do not double the next dose.

STOPPING THE DRUG
Take the prescription-strength medication for the full treatment period, even if you begin to feel better before the scheduled end of therapy.

PROLONGED USE
Do not take the OTC non-prescription-strength drug for more than 2 weeks unless you have been otherwise instructed by your doctor.

▼ PRECAUTIONS

Over 60: Adverse reactions may be more likely and more severe in older patients.

Driving and Hazardous Work: Do not drive or engage in hazardous work until you determine how the medicine affects you.

Alcohol: Avoid alcoholic beverages. Ranitidine may increase blood alcohol levels.

Pregnancy: Risks vary, depending on the patient and dosage. Consult your doctor.

Breast Feeding: Ranitidine passes into breast milk and may pose harm to the child; avoid or discontinue use while nursing.

Infants and Children: Ranitidine is not recommended for young patients, although it has not been shown to cause any side effects or problems different from those in adults when used for short periods of time.

Special Concerns: Avoid cigarette smoking because it may increase stomach acid secretion and thus worsen the disease. Do not take ranitidine if you have ever had an allergic reaction to a histamine (H2) blocker. If stomach pain becomes worse while using the drug, be sure to tell your doctor right away.

OVERDOSE
Symptoms: Vomiting, diarrhea, breathing problems, slurred speech, rapid heartbeat, delirium.

What to Do: Call your doctor, emergency medical services (EMS), or the nearest poison control center immediately.

▼ INTERACTIONS

DRUG INTERACTIONS
Consult your doctor for specific advice if you are taking antacids, antidepressants, aspirin, beta-blockers, caffeine, diazepam, glipizide, ketoconazole, lidocaine, phenytoin, procainamide, theophylline, or warfarin.

FOOD INTERACTIONS
Carbonated drinks, citrus fruits and juices, caffeine-containing beverages, and other acidic foods or liquids may irritate the stomach or interfere with the therapeutic action of ranitidine.

DISEASE INTERACTIONS
Patients with kidney disease should not use ranitidine or should use it in smaller, limited doses under careful supervision by a physician.

≡ SIDE EFFECTS ≡

SERIOUS
Irregular heart rhythm (palpitations), slowed heartbeat, severe blood problems resulting in unusual bleeding, bruising, fever, chills, and increased susceptibility to infection. Call your doctor immediately.

COMMON
Headache, fatigue, drowsiness, dizziness, nausea, vomiting, abdominal pain, diarrhea, constipation.

LESS COMMON
Blurred vision, decreased sexual desire or function, swelling of breasts in males or females, temporary hair loss, hallucinations, depression, insomnia, skin rash, hives, or redness.

RESORCINOL

BRAND NAMES

Acnomel Cream, Clearasil Adult Stick, RA Lotion, Rezamid Acne Lotion

Available in: Lotion, cream, stick
Available as Generic? Yes
Drug Class: Acne drug

▼ USAGE INFORMATION

WHY IT'S TAKEN
To treat acne and seborrheic dermatitis. Resorcinol is also infrequently used to treat eczema, psoriasis, corns, calluses, warts, and other similar skin conditions.

HOW IT WORKS
Resorcinol fights fungal and bacterial organisms that can cause infection and promotes the softening, dissolution, and peeling of the skin.

▼ DOSAGE GUIDELINES

RANGE AND FREQUENCY
For acne and seborrheic dermatitis: Apply once or twice daily as recommended or as tolerated. Wash your hands thoroughly after each application of resorcinol.

ONSET OF EFFECT
Unknown.

DURATION OF ACTION
Unknown.

DIETARY ADVICE
No special restrictions.

STORAGE
Store in a tightly sealed container away from heat and direct light.

MISSED DOSE
Skip the missed application and resume your regular dosage schedule. Do not double the next dose.

STOPPING THE DRUG
If you are using resorcinol on doctor's orders, the decision to stop using the drug should be made by your doctor. If you are using the drug without a prescription, you may stop using it whenever your acne clears; however, it is likely that discontinuing use of the drug will lead to a recurrence of acne.

PROLONGED USE
Do not use resorcinol for longer than prescribed.

▼ PRECAUTIONS

Over 60:
No special advice.

Driving and Hazardous Work:
No special precautions are necessary.

Alcohol:
No special precautions are necessary.

Pregnancy:
Resorcinol has not been shown to cause birth defects or other problems during pregnancy. It may, however, be absorbed through the skin. Consult your doctor for specific advice if you are pregnant or plan to become pregnant.

Breast Feeding:
Resorcinol may be absorbed into the body through the skin; caution is advised. Consult your doctor for advice.

Infants and Children:
Youngsters should not use resorcinol on large areas of the body.

Special Concerns:
Anyone with a history of allergy to resorcinol or any other ingredients in the specific product should not use this medication. Resorcinol should not be used on wounds, because it may cause methemoglobinemia, a blood disorder. It should not be applied over large areas of the body, especially when it is used in high concentrations. Avoid contact of resorcinol with the eyes. This medication is generally not recommended for black persons, since it may significantly darken treated areas of skin. Resorcinol may darken light-colored hair.

OVERDOSE
Symptoms: If ingested, diarrhea, nausea, abdominal pain, vomiting, drowsiness, dizziness, severe or persistent headache, breathing difficulty, unusual tiredness or weakness, slow heartbeat, and profuse sweating may occur.

What to Do: In case of resorcinol ingestion, call your doctor, emergency medical services (EMS), or the nearest poison control center.

▼ INTERACTIONS

DRUG INTERACTIONS
The following drugs or other products may irritate the skin and therefore should not be used with resorcinol unless recommended by your doctor: abrasive cleansers or soaps, alcohol-containing preparations (including astringents, aftershave lotions, other perfumed toiletries), any other acne agent, any preparation containing a peeling agent such as benzoyl peroxide, salicylic acid, alpha hydroxy acids, sulfur, or vitamin A, and soaps, medicated cosmetics, or other cosmetics that dry the skin.

FOOD INTERACTIONS
No known food interactions.

DISEASE INTERACTIONS
You should not use resorcinol if you have had a prior allergic reaction to it.

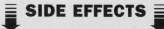

≣ SIDE EFFECTS ≣

SERIOUS
No serious side effects are associated with resorcinol during normal use (as prescribed).

COMMON
Mild redness and peeling of the skin. Such side effects tend to occur at the beginning of therapy and diminish as your body adjusts to the medication; notify your doctor if such symptoms persist or interfere with daily activities.

LESS COMMON
More-severe irritation or allergy with redness, peeling, burning, stinging, itching, or rash. Call your doctor.

SENNA

Available in: Tablets, granules, oral solution, syrup
Available as Generic? No
Drug Class: Laxative

BRAND NAMES

Black-Draught Lax-Senna, Correctol Herbal Tea, Dosaflex, Dr. Caldwell Senna Laxative, Ex-Lax, Fletcher's Castoria, Senexon, Senna-Gen, Senokot, Senolax, X-Prep Liquid

▼ USAGE INFORMATION

WHY IT'S TAKEN
For short-term treatment of constipation.

HOW IT WORKS
Senna stimulates water and electrolyte (mineral salt) secretion in the intestine to induce defecation.

▼ DOSAGE GUIDELINES

RANGE AND FREQUENCY
Adults and teenagers: 2 tablets, or 1 teaspoon of granules, or 10 to 15 ml of syrup. Children ages 6 to 12: 1 tablet or ½ teaspoon of granules. Take at bedtime.

ONSET OF EFFECT
Within 6 to 10 hours.

DURATION OF ACTION
Variable.

DIETARY ADVICE
Each dose of senna should be taken on an empty stomach with 8 oz of water or fruit juice.

STORAGE
Store in a tightly sealed container away from moisture, heat, and direct light.

MISSED DOSE
Take it as soon as you remember. If it is near the time for the next dose, skip the missed dose and resume your regular dosage schedule. Do not double the next dose.

STOPPING THE DRUG
Take senna as directed for the full treatment period. You may stop taking the drug if you are feeling better before the scheduled end of therapy.

PROLONGED USE
If regular bowel movement does not resume in 1 week, discontinue use of senna and consult your doctor.

▼ PRECAUTIONS

Over 60: Adverse reactions may be more likely and more severe in older patients.

Driving and Hazardous Work: Do not drive or engage in hazardous work until you determine how the medicine affects you.

Alcohol: Avoid alcohol.

Pregnancy: Senna may cause unwanted effects during pregnancy if not used properly. Consult your doctor.

Breast Feeding: Senna may pass into breast milk; caution is advised. Consult your doctor for advice.

Infants and Children: Senna is not recommended for use by children under the age of 6 unless it has been prescribed by a doctor.

Special Concerns: You should increase your intake of foods containing vitamin D, such as milk products, and maintain an adequate intake of foods containing folic acid, such as fresh vegetables, fruits, whole grains, and liver, while taking senna. Senna is one of the most effective laxatives for relieving the severe constipation caused by narcotic analgesics like morphine and codeine.

OVERDOSE
Symptoms: Sudden vomiting, nausea, diarrhea, or cramping.

What to Do: An overdose of senna is unlikely to be life-threatening. However, if someone takes a much larger dose than prescribed, call your doctor, emergency medical services (EMS), or the nearest poison control center immediately.

▼ INTERACTIONS

DRUG INTERACTIONS
Do not take any other medicine within 2 hours of taking senna. Consult your doctor for specific advice if you are taking anticoagulants, digitalis drugs, ciprofloxacin, etidronate, sodium poly-styrene sulfonate, or oral tetracycline antibiotics.

FOOD INTERACTIONS
No known food interactions.

DISEASE INTERACTIONS
Use caution when taking senna. Consult your doctor if you have a history of any of the following: appendicitis, rectal bleeding of unknown cause, colostomy, intestinal blockage, ileostomy, diabetes, heart disease, high blood pressure, kidney disease, or difficulty swallowing.

⟱ SIDE EFFECTS ⟱

SERIOUS
Confusion, irregular heartbeat, muscle cramps, pink to red or yellow to brown coloration of urine and stools, unusual tiredness or weakness, laxative dependence. Call your doctor immediately.

COMMON
Belching, cramping, diarrhea, nausea.

LESS COMMON
No less-common side effects have been reported.

SIMETHICONE

Available in: Tablets, chewable tablets, capsules, drops
Available as Generic? Yes
Drug Class: Antacid; antiflatulant

▼ USAGE INFORMATION

WHY IT'S TAKEN
To relieve pain caused by excess gas in stomach and intestines. It may also be employed in a clinical setting to decrease gas before diagnostic radiography of the stomach or intestines, or prior to endoscopy.

HOW IT WORKS
Simethicone disperses throughout the gastrointestinal tract and prevents the formation of gas bubbles.

▼ DOSAGE GUIDELINES

RANGE AND FREQUENCY
Tablets or capsules: 60 to 125 mg, 4 times a day, after meals and at bedtime. Chewable tablets: 40 to 125 mg, 4 times a day after meals and at bedtime, or 150 mg, 3 times a day after meals. Drops: Take 40 to 95 mg by mouth, 4 times a day after meals and at bedtime. The dose should not exceed 500 mg a day for all forms unless your doctor advises otherwise.

ONSET OF EFFECT
Immediate.

DURATION OF ACTION
Unknown.

DIETARY ADVICE
This medicine should be taken after meals and at bedtime for optimal results.

STORAGE
Store in a tightly sealed container away from heat, moisture, and direct light. Store the liquid form at room temperature.

MISSED DOSE
Take it as soon as you remember. However, if it is near the time for the next dose, skip the missed dose and resume your regular dosage schedule. Do not double the next dose.

STOPPING THE DRUG
Take simethicone as recommended for the full treatment period. However, you may stop taking the drug if you are feeling better before the scheduled end of therapy.

PROLONGED USE
Consult your doctor if you take simethicone for a prolonged period.

▼ PRECAUTIONS

Over 60: There is no specific information comparing use of simethicone in older persons with use in younger persons.

However, no special problems are expected.

Driving and Hazardous Work: The use of simithicone should not impair your ability to perform such tasks safely.

Alcohol: No special problems are expected.

Pregnancy: Simethicone is not absorbed into the body and is not expected to cause problems during pregnancy.

Breast Feeding: Simethicone has not been reported to cause problems in babies who are nursed.

Infants and Children: Use of simethicone for the treatment of infant colic is not recommended because of limited information on its safety in infants. Simethicone should be given to children only under a doctor's instructions.

Special Concerns: If you take the chewable tablets, chew them thoroughly before swallowing for more complete and faster results. Shake the liquid form well before using. You should change position frequently and walk about to help eliminate gas. Tell your doctor if you are on a low-sodium, low-sugar, or other special diet. You should exercise regularly and develop regular bowel habits. Do not smoke before meals.

OVERDOSE
Symptoms: No specific ones have been reported.

What to Do: An overdose of simethicone is not life-threatening. However, if someone takes a much larger

dose than recommended, call your doctor or the nearest poison control center.

▼ INTERACTIONS

DRUG INTERACTIONS
None known.

FOOD INTERACTIONS
Avoid any foods that increase gas formation. Chew your food slowly and thoroughly. Avoid carbonated drinks.

DISEASE INTERACTIONS
None known.

≣ SIDE EFFECTS ≣

SERIOUS
No serious side effects have been reported.

COMMON
Expulsion of excess gas causing belching and flatulence.

LESS COMMON
No less-common side effects have been reported.

SODIUM BICARBONATE

Available in: Effervescent powder, powder, tablets
Available as Generic? Yes
Drug Class: Antacid

▼ USAGE INFORMATION

WHY IT'S TAKEN
To relieve heartburn, sour stomach, or acid indigestion. It may also be prescribed to treat metabolic acidosis (excess acid buildup in the body fluids), to prevent urinary stones, and as part of the treatment of gout.

HOW IT WORKS
Sodium bicarbonate neutralizes stomach acid and reduces the action of pepsin, a digestive enzyme. This provides symptomatic relief from excess stomach acid. Also, the bicarbonate is a base, meaning it can help correct the pH balance (reduce the acidity) of blood and urine.

▼ DOSAGE GUIDELINES

RANGE AND FREQUENCY
Effervescent powder—For heartburn or sour stomach: 3.9 to 10 g (1 to 2½ teaspoons) in a glass of cold water. Usually not more than 19.5 g a day (5 teaspoons). Children ages 6 to 12: 1 to 1.9 g (¼ to ½ teaspoon) in a glass of cold water. Powder—For heartburn or sour stomach: ½ teaspoon in a glass of water every 2 hours. Dose may be changed if needed. To make the urine less acidic: 1 teaspoon (1.9 g) in a glass of water every 4 hours; usually not more than 4 teaspoons a day. Dose may be changed by your doctor. Tablets—For heartburn or sour stomach: 325 mg to 2 g, 1 to 4 times a day. Children ages 6 to 12: 520 mg. Dose may be repeated in 30 minutes. To make the urine less acidic—To start, 4 g; then 1 to 2 g every 4 hours. Maximum adult dose usually not more than 16 g a day. Children: 23 to 230 mg per 2.2 lbs (1 kg) of body weight a day. The dose may be changed if needed.

ONSET OF EFFECT
Rapid when used as an antacid for heartburn and sour stomach.

DURATION OF ACTION
Unknown.

DIETARY ADVICE
Sodium bicarbonate should be taken after meals. Be sure to account for the large amount of sodium in this medication if you are on a salt-restricted diet.

STORAGE
Store in a tightly sealed container away from moisture, heat, and direct light.

MISSED DOSE
Take it as soon as you remember. If it is near the time for the next dose, skip the missed dose and resume your regular dosage schedule. Do not double the next dose.

STOPPING THE DRUG
Take as directed if taking it by prescription.

PROLONGED USE
Do not take sodium bicarbonate for more than 2 weeks or on a routine basis without consulting your physician about its use.

▼ PRECAUTIONS

Over 60: See Dietary Advice.

Driving and Hazardous Work: No special precautions are necessary.

Alcohol: Avoid alcohol.

Pregnancy: No problems have been reported.

Breast Feeding: No problems have been reported.

Infants and Children: Use and dosage for infants and children under 6 years of age should be determined by your doctor.

OVERDOSE
Symptoms: See Serious Side Effects.

What to Do: An overdose of sodium bicarbonate is unlikely to be life-threatening. However, if someone takes a much larger dose than recommended, call your doctor, emergency medical services (EMS), or the nearest poison control center immediately.

▼ INTERACTIONS

DRUG INTERACTIONS
Do not take more than one OTC medication containing sodium bicarbonate at a time. Consult your doctor for specific advice if you are taking ketoconazole, tetracyclines, mecamylamine, methenamine, urinary acidifiers, amphetamines, anticholinergics, quinidine, citrates, enteric-coated medications, ephedrine, flecainide, fluoroquinolones, iron, lithium, methotrexate, mexiletine, sucralfate, or salicylates.

FOOD INTERACTIONS
Do not take sodium bicarbonate with milk or milk products.

DISEASE INTERACTIONS
Do not take sodium bicarbonate if you are experiencing any sign of appendicitis (stomach pain, bloating, nausea, and vomiting). If you have any kidney problems, use sodium bicarbonate only on advice of your doctor. Consult your doctor if you have intestinal or rectal bleeding, edema (swelling of the hands or feet), heart, liver, or kidney disease, hypertension, urination problems, or preeclampsia during pregnancy.

≣ SIDE EFFECTS ≣

SERIOUS
Frequent urge to urinate, nervousness or restlessness, mental or mood changes, muscle twitching or pain, nausea or vomiting, slow breathing, continuing headache, loss of appetite, swelling of feet or lower legs, unpleasant taste, unusual fatigue. Call your doctor immediately.

COMMON
No common side effects have been reported.

LESS COMMON
Stomach cramps, increased thirst.

SODIUM PHOSPHATE/SODIUM BIPHOSPHATE

Available in: Oral solution, effervescent powder, enema
Available as Generic? Yes
Drug Class: Hyperosmotic laxative

▼ USAGE INFORMATION

WHY IT'S TAKEN
To treat short-term constipation or for rapid emptying of the colon prior to bowel or rectal examination.

HOW IT WORKS
This medication attracts and retains water in the intestine, increasing peristalsis (bowel activity) and creating the urge to defecate.

▼ DOSAGE GUIDELINES

RANGE AND FREQUENCY
Oral–Adults and teenagers: 20 to 30 ml (4 to 6 teaspoons) mixed with ½ glass cool water. Children ages 10 to 12: 10 ml (2 teaspoons). Children ages 6 to 10: 5 ml (1 teaspoon). Enema–Adults and teenagers: 118 ml (contents of 1 disposable adult enema) given rectally. Children over 2: ½ adult dose (entire contents of 1 disposable pediatric enema).

ONSET OF EFFECT
30 minutes to 3 hours after oral administration, 3 to 5 minutes after enema.

DURATION OF ACTION
Variable with oral use; upon evacuation with enema.

DIETARY ADVICE
Sodium phosphate/sodium biphosphate should not be used with food. The unpleasant taste that may occur when you take the medicine can be lessened by taking it with citrus fruit juice or a citrus-flavored soft drink.

STORAGE
Store in a tightly sealed container away from heat and direct light.

MISSED DOSE
Oral forms: If you are taking this laxative on a fixed schedule, take the missed dose as soon as you remember. If it is near the time for the next dose, skip the missed dose and resume your regular dosage schedule. Do not double the next dose. Enema: Not applicable.

STOPPING THE DRUG
Take the medicine as directed for the full treatment period. You may stop taking the drug, however, if you feel better before the scheduled end of therapy.

PROLONGED USE
Do not use any laxative for longer than 2 weeks without consulting your doctor.

▼ PRECAUTIONS

Over 60: Adverse reactions may be more likely and more severe in older patients.

Driving and Hazardous Work: Do not drive or engage in hazardous work until you determine how the medicine affects you.

Alcohol: Avoid alcohol.

Pregnancy: This laxative contains a large amount of sodium, which may have unwanted effects during pregnancy, such as higher blood pressure. If you have to take a laxative during pregnancy, consult your doctor for specific advice.

Breast Feeding: Sodium phosphate may pass into breast milk; caution is advised. Consult your doctor for specific advice.

Infants and Children: Do not give sodium phosphate/sodium biphosphate to a child under the age of 6 without consulting your doctor.

Special Concerns: Chilling the oral form of the medication or taking it with ice or following it with citrus fruit juice or citrus-flavored carbonated beverages may make it more palatable. Remember that chronic use of sodium phosphate or any laxative can lead to laxative dependence. You should consume adequate amounts of bulk (fiber) in your diet, such as bran, whole-grain cereals, fruit, and vegetables. This laxative should be taken on a schedule that does not interfere with activities or sleep; it produces watery stools within 3 to 6 hours. It should not be taken within 2 hours of taking other medications.

OVERDOSE
Symptoms: Excessive bowel activity, dehydration causing low blood pressure and abnormal heartbeat, metabolic acidosis, blood chemistry abnormalities.

What to Do: An overdose of sodium phosphate/sodium biphosphate is unlikely to be life-threatening. However, if someone takes a much larger dose than prescribed, call your doctor, emergency medical services (EMS), or the nearest poison control center immediately.

▼ INTERACTIONS

DRUG INTERACTIONS
Consult your doctor for advice if you are taking anticoagulants, digitalis drugs, ciprofloxacin, etidronate, sodium polystyrene sulfonate, or oral tetracyclines.

FOOD INTERACTIONS
No known food interactions.

DISEASE INTERACTIONS
Consult your doctor if you have a history of appendicitis, rectal bleeding of unknown cause, colostomy, intestinal blockage, ileostomy, diabetes mellitus, heart disease, high blood pressure, kidney disease, or any difficulties in swallowing.

≡ SIDE EFFECTS ≡

SERIOUS
Confusion, dizziness or lightheadedness, irregular heartbeat, muscle cramps, unusual tiredness or weakness. Call your doctor immediately.

COMMON
Cramping, diarrhea, gas, increased thirst.

LESS COMMON
No less-common side effects have been reported.

SULFUR TOPICAL

BRAND NAMES

Cuticura Ointment, Finac, Fostex Regular Strength Medicated Cover-Up, Fostril Lotion, Lotio-Asulfa, Sulpho-Lac

Available in: Cream, lotion, ointment, bar soap
Available as Generic? Yes
Drug Class: Acne drug

▼ USAGE INFORMATION

WHY IT'S TAKEN
To treat skin conditions including acne, seborrheic dermatitis, and scabies.

HOW IT WORKS
Topical sulfur is lethal to various strains of bacteria (which are a primary cause of acne), fungus, parasites, and other types of microorganisms. It also promotes softening, dissolution, and peeling of hard, scaly, roughened, or irregular surface skin.

▼ DOSAGE GUIDELINES

RANGE AND FREQUENCY
For acne, lotion, cream, or bar soap: Use on skin as needed. To use the soap, work up a rich lather using warm water. Wash the affected area, rinse thoroughly, apply again and rub in gently for a few minutes. Remove excess lather with a towel or tissue, without rinsing. Lotion: Apply 2 or 3 times a day. Ointment: Apply the 0.5% ointment as needed. Wash the affected area with soap and water and dry thoroughly before application. For seborrheic dermatitis: Use 1 or 2 times a day as directed on the package instructions. For scabies: Apply the 6% ointment every night for 3 nights. The ointment should be applied to the entire body from the neck down. You may bathe before each application and should bathe 24 hours after the last (third) application.

ONSET OF EFFECT
Unknown.

DURATION OF ACTION
Unknown.

DIETARY ADVICE
Topical sulfur can be used without regard to diet.

STORAGE
Store in a tightly sealed container away from heat and direct light. Keep the cream, lotion, and ointment forms from freezing.

MISSED DOSE
Resume your regular dosage schedule with the next application. Do not double the next dose.

STOPPING THE DRUG
If you are using sulfur by prescription, the decision to stop taking the drug should be made by your doctor. If you are using it without a prescription, you may stop taking the drug when your skin has cleared; however, it is likely that the condition will recur.

PROLONGED USE
If your doctor recommends sulfur, use it no longer than directed.

▼ PRECAUTIONS

Over 60: No special precautions required.

Driving and Hazardous Work: No special precautions are necessary.

Alcohol: No special precautions are necessary.

Pregnancy: Sulfur has not been shown to cause birth defects or other problems during pregnancy. Before you use sulfur, tell your doctor if you are pregnant or plan to become pregnant.

Breast Feeding: Topical sulfur has not been reported to cause problems in nursing infants. Consult your doctor for specific advice.

Infants and Children: Use and dosage for children must be determined by your pediatrician.

Special Concerns: Anyone with a history of allergy to sulfur and other ingredients in the medication should not use this product. Keep sulfur away from the eyes. If you accidentally get some of the medicine in your eyes, flush them thoroughly with water.

▼ OVERDOSE

Symptoms: Excessive application of topical sulfur may lead to more severe irritation of the skin.

What to Do: If topical sulfur is accidentally ingested, call your doctor, emergency medical services (EMS), or the nearest poison control center immediately.

▼ INTERACTIONS

DRUG INTERACTIONS
Consult your doctor for specific advice if you are using abrasive soaps or cleansers, alcohol-containing preparations, any other acne agent, any preparation containing a peeling agent such as benzoyl peroxide, salicylic acid, alpha hydroxy acids, sulfur, or vitamin A, or soaps, medicated cosmetics, or other cosmetics that dry the skin. Also tell your doctor if you are using any other prescription or over-the-counter drug for a skin condition.

FOOD INTERACTIONS
No known food interactions.

DISEASE INTERACTIONS
You should not use sulfur if you have had a prior allergic reaction to it.

≡ SIDE EFFECTS ≡

SERIOUS
No serious side effects have been reported.

COMMON
Mild redness and peeling of skin.

LESS COMMON
Skin irritation or allergy with redness, peeling, burning, stinging, itching, or rash. Contact your doctor.

TERBINAFINE HYDROCHLORIDE

Available in: Topical cream
Available as Generic? No
Drug Class: Antifungal

▼ USAGE INFORMATION

WHY IT'S TAKEN
The cream is used to treat fungal infections of the skin, such as tinea corporis (ringworm), tinea cruris (jock itch), and tinea pedis (athlete's foot).

HOW IT WORKS
Terbinafine inhibits an enzyme essential for the production of substances vital for the reproduction and survival of some types of fungal organisms.

▼ DOSAGE GUIDELINES

RANGE AND FREQUENCY
Apply a thin film of medicine to the affected area 1 to 2 times a day for ringworm or jock itch; 2 times a day for athlete's foot. Apply the cream for at least 1 week, but no longer than 4 weeks.

ONSET OF EFFECT
Unknown.

DURATION OF ACTION
Unknown.

DIETARY ADVICE
Terbinafine can be applied without regard to meals.

STORAGE
Store in a tightly sealed container away from moisture, heat, and direct light. Do not allow the cream to freeze.

MISSED DOSE
It is important to not miss any doses. Apply as soon as you remember. If you do not remember until the next day, skip the missed dose and resume your regular dosage schedule. Do not use excessive amounts of the cream.

STOPPING THE DRUG
Use for as long as directed or until infection clears.

PROLONGED USE
Side effects are more likely to occur with prolonged use.

▼ PRECAUTIONS

Over 60: No special advice.

Driving and Hazardous Work: No special precautions.

Alcohol: No special warnings.

Pregnancy: Not recommended for pregnant women.

Breast Feeding: Avoid while nursing.

Infants and Children: Terbinafine is not recommended for children under the age of 18.

Special Concerns: Wash your hands before and after applying the cream. Avoid allowing topical terbinafine to come into contact with the eyes, nose, and mouth. If using terbinafine for ringworm, wear loose-fitting, well-ventilated clothing and avoid excess heat and humidity. It is also recommended to use a bland, absorbent powder like talcum once or twice a day after the cream has been applied and absorbed by the skin. If using the medication for jock itch, do not wear underwear that is tight or made from synthetic materials; wear loose-fitting cotton underwear. If using terbinafine for athlete's foot, dry your feet carefully after bathing and wear clean cotton socks with sandals or well-ventilated shoes. Before applying the medication, wash the affected area with soap and warm water and dry thoroughly.

OVERDOSE
Symptoms: An overdose with terbinafine cream is unlikely.

What to Do: Call your doctor as soon as possible.

▼ INTERACTIONS

DRUG INTERACTIONS
Consult your doctor if you are using any other preparation that is to be applied to the same area of skin as terbinafine cream.

FOOD INTERACTIONS
No known food interactions.

DISEASE INTERACTIONS
No disease interactions have been reported.

≡ SIDE EFFECTS ≡

SERIOUS
Serious side effects with terbinafine are rare. However, terbinafine tablets may cause liver dysfunction; severe skin reactions such as Stevens-Johnson syndrome; severe blood disorders, potentially resulting in increased susceptibility to infection, uncontrolled bleeding or other problems; or severe allergic reactions. Seek emergency medical assistance immediately.

COMMON
Headache, diarrhea, rash, stomach pain, indigestion, nausea.

LESS COMMON
Tablets may cause flatulence, itching, skin eruptions, loss of taste, weakness, fatigue, vomiting, joint and muscle pain, or hair loss. Terbinafine cream may cause redness, itching, burning, blistering, swelling, oozing, or other signs of skin irritation not present before using the drug.

TIOCONAZOLE

Available in: Vaginal ointment
Available as Generic? No
Drug Class: Antifungal

▼ USAGE INFORMATION

WHY IT'S TAKEN
To treat fungal (yeast) infections of the vagina.

HOW IT WORKS
Tioconazole prevents the growth and function of some fungal organisms by interfering with the production of substances needed to preserve the cell membrane. This drug is effective only for infections caused by fungal organisms. It will not work for bacterial or viral infections.

▼ DOSAGE GUIDELINES

RANGE AND FREQUENCY
A single 300 mg (1 applicatorful) dose of ointment, inserted with an applicator into the vagina at bedtime.

ONSET OF EFFECT
Some relief may be felt within 1 day. Complete relief of symptoms generally occurs within 7 days.

DURATION OF ACTION
Unknown.

DIETARY ADVICE
Tioconazole may be used without regard to diet.

STORAGE
Store in a tightly sealed container away from moisture, heat, and direct light. Do not allow it to freeze.

MISSED DOSE
Not applicable. Tioconazole is usually effective with a single, one-time use.

STOPPING THE DRUG
Tioconazole is generally used on a one-time basis. If needed, a second dose may be applied 1 to 2 weeks following the first dose.

PROLONGED USE
Tioconazole is for short-term use only.

▼ PRECAUTIONS

Over 60: No special problems are expected.

Driving and Hazardous Work: This drug should not impair your ability to perform such tasks safely.

Alcohol: No special warnings.

Pregnancy: Adequate studies on the use of tioconazole during pregnancy have not been done; however, there are no reports of adverse effects while using it. Consult your doctor before using.

Breast Feeding: No problems are expected. Consult your doctor before using this medicine while nursing.

Infants and Children: No studies have been done on the use of tioconazole in children. Consult a pediatrician for specific advice.

Special Concerns: Tioconazole may be used with oral contraceptives and antibiotic therapy. Sanitary napkins should be used to prevent staining of clothing. The affected area should be kept cool and dry. The patient should wear loose-fitting cotton clothing and freshly laundered cotton underwear or pantyhose with a cotton crotch. Avoid underwear made from nonventilating materials. Do not sit for a long time in a wet bathing suit. Avoid feminine hygiene sprays. Wash daily with unscented soap and dry thoroughly with a clean towel. Tampons should not be used during therapy. Do not have sex for 3 days after treatment and wait an additional 3 days before relying upon a condom or diaphragm, since the medication may weaken latex. After this time, the patient's sexual partner should wear a condom during intercourse and should consult a doctor if penile redness, itching, or discomfort occurs. You may use this medicine during your menstrual period. After urination or a bowel movement, cleanse by wiping the area from front to back to prevent reinfection by yeast.

OVERDOSE
Symptoms: An overdose with tioconazole is unlikely.

What to Do: If someone should swallow a large amount of the medicine, call the doctor.

▼ INTERACTIONS

DRUG INTERACTIONS
Tell your doctor if you are using any other OTC or prescription vaginal medication.

FOOD INTERACTIONS
No food interactions have been reported.

DISEASE INTERACTIONS
No disease interactions have been reported.

⩘ SIDE EFFECTS ⩘

SERIOUS
Vaginal itching, burning, discharge, or irritation not present prior to treatment. Call your doctor as soon as possible.

COMMON
No common side effects have been reported.

LESS COMMON
Headache, stomach cramps or pain, irritation or burning of sexual partner's penis.

TOLNAFTATE

Available in: Cream, gel, powder, solution
Available as Generic? Yes
Drug Class: Topical antifungal

▼ USAGE INFORMATION

WHY IT'S TAKEN
To treat a variety of fungal infections of the skin, including tinea corporis (ringworm), tinea cruris (jock itch), and tinea pedis (athlete's foot).

HOW IT WORKS
Tolnaftate prevents fungi from manufacturing vital substances required for growth and function. This medication is effective only for infections caused by ringworm fungal organisms. It will not work for bacterial or viral infections.

▼ DOSAGE GUIDELINES

RANGE AND FREQUENCY
Apply to the affected area 2 times a day. All forms should be used immediately after the affected area is washed and dried. Wash your hands before and after application.

ONSET OF EFFECT
Unknown.

DURATION OF ACTION
Unknown.

DIETARY ADVICE
No special restrictions.

STORAGE
Store in a tightly sealed container away from moisture, heat, and direct light.

MISSED DOSE
Apply it as soon as you remember. If it is near the time for the next dose, skip the missed dose and resume your regular dosage schedule. Do not double the next dose.

STOPPING THE DRUG
Use of tolnaftate should continue for 2 weeks beyond the time that symptoms disappear. This helps to ensure eradication of the fungus.

PROLONGED USE
You should consult your doctor if symptoms do not improve within 10 days of beginning therapy.

▼ PRECAUTIONS

Over 60: No special problems are expected.

Driving and Hazardous Work: The use of tolnaftate should not impair your ability to perform such tasks safely.

Alcohol: No special warnings.

Pregnancy: Tolnaftate has not been shown in studies to cause problems when used during pregnancy.

Breast Feeding: Tolnaftate may pass into breast milk, but no problems have been reported. Consult your doctor for specific advice.

Infants and Children: Children younger than age 2 should use tolnaftate only under the close supervision of a pediatrician.

Special Concerns: Do not allow tolnaftate to come into contact with your eyes. If your skin condition does not improve or instead gets worse after 10 days of treatment, consult your doctor. Tolnaftate should not be used alone to treat fungal infections of the hair or nails; your doctor can prescribe an additional medication for this condition. If you are using tolnaftate for an infection of the feet, be sure to wear well-fitting and well-ventilated shoes and to change your shoes and put on clean socks every day. Do not cover the treated area of skin with bandages unless your doctor specifically instructs you to do so.

OVERDOSE
Symptoms: None are known; no cases of overdose have been reported.

What to Do: An overdose of tolnaftate is unlikely to occur. However, if someone accidentally ingests some of the medication, call your doctor, emergency medical services (EMS), or the nearest poison control center immediately.

▼ INTERACTIONS

DRUG INTERACTIONS
Some drugs may interact adversely with tolnaftate. Consult your doctor for specific advice if you are using any other prescription or OTC medication that is applied to the same area of skin being treated by tolnaftate.

FOOD INTERACTIONS
No known food interactions.

DISEASE INTERACTIONS
Caution is advised when taking tolnaftate. Consult your doctor for specific advice if you have a history of any other skin condition.

≡ SIDE EFFECTS ≡

SERIOUS
Skin irritation that was not present before use of tolnaftate. Call your doctor immediately.

COMMON
No common side effects are associated with the use of tolnaftate.

LESS COMMON
No less-common side effects are associated with the use of tolnaftate.

TRIPROLIDINE HYDROCHLORIDE

Available in: Syrup
Available as Generic? Yes
Drug Class: Antihistamine

▼ USAGE INFORMATION

WHY IT'S TAKEN
To relieve symptoms of hay fever and other allergies.

HOW IT WORKS
Triprolidine blocks the effects of histamine, a naturally occurring substance that causes swelling, itching, sneezing, watery eyes, hives, and other symptoms of allergic reaction.

▼ DOSAGE GUIDELINES

RANGE AND FREQUENCY
Adults and children age 12 and over: 2.5 mg every 4 to 6 hours. The maximum dose is 10 mg per day. Children ages 6 to 12: 1.25 mg (1 teaspoon) every 4 to 6 hours. The maximum dose is 5 mg per day. Children ages 4 to 6: 0.938 mg (¾ teaspoon) every 4 to 6 hours. The maximum dose is 3.744 mg per day. Children ages 2 to 4: 0.625 mg (½ teaspoon) every 4 to 6 hours. The maximum dose is 2.5 mg per day. Children ages 4 months to 2 years: 0.313 mg (¼ teaspoon) every 4 to 6 hours. The maximum dose is 1.25 mg per day.

ONSET OF EFFECT
15 to 60 minutes.

DURATION OF ACTION
4 to 6 hours.

DIETARY ADVICE
Take with food or milk to reduce stomach upset.

STORAGE
Store in a tightly sealed container away from heat and direct light. Do not allow the drug to freeze.

MISSED DOSE
Take it as soon as you remember. If it is near the time for the next dose, skip the missed dose and resume your regular dosage schedule. Do not double the next dose.

STOPPING THE DRUG
The decision to stop taking the drug should be made by your doctor.

PROLONGED USE
Tolerance, or decreased responsiveness to the drug, usually does not develop with prolonged use. If it does, consult your doctor.

▼ PRECAUTIONS

Over 60: Adverse reactions may be more likely and more severe in older patients.

Driving and Hazardous Work: Do not drive or engage in hazardous work until you determine how the medicine affects you.

Alcohol: Avoid alcohol.

Pregnancy: Before you take triprolidine, tell your doctor if you are pregnant or plan to become pregnant.

Breast Feeding: Triprolidine passes into breast milk; avoid or discontinue use while nursing. Flow of breast milk may be reduced.

Infants and Children: Adverse effects may be more likely to occur and be more severe in children.

Special Concerns: Stop taking triprolidine 4 days before you have an allergy skin test. Drink water frequently or use ice chips, sugarless candy, or sugarless gum if dry mouth occurs. Coffee or tea may reduce the common side effect of drowsiness.

OVERDOSE
Symptoms: Central nervous system depression or, paradoxically, nervous system stimulation; very low blood pressure; breathing difficulty; seizures; loss of consciousness; severe dryness of the mouth, nose, or throat.

What to Do: Call your doctor, emergency medical services (EMS), or the nearest poison control center immediately.

▼ INTERACTIONS

DRUG INTERACTIONS
Consult your doctor for advice if you are taking anticholinergics, clarithromycin, erythromycin, itraconazole, ketoconazole, bepridil, disopyramide, maprotiline, phenothiazines, pimozide, procainamide, quinidine, tricyclic antidepressants, central nervous system depressants, MAO inhibitors, or quinine.

FOOD INTERACTIONS
No known food interactions.

DISEASE INTERACTIONS
Caution is advised when taking triprolidine. Consult your doctor if you have an enlarged prostate, urinary tract blockage, difficulty in urinating, or glaucoma. Use of triprolidine may cause complications in patients with liver disease, since this organ works to remove the medication from the body.

≡ SIDE EFFECTS ≡

SERIOUS
Sore throat and fever, unusual tiredness or weakness, unusual bleeding or bruising. Call your doctor immediately.

COMMON
Drowsiness, thickening of mucus.

LESS COMMON
Blurred vision; rapid heartbeat; skin rash; stomach upset; nervousness; increased sensitivity of skin to sunlight; confusion; difficult or painful urination; dizziness; dry mouth, nose, or throat; loss of appetite; nightmares; ringing or buzzing in ears; restlessness; irritability.

UNDECYLENIC ACID

Available in: Aerosol foam, aerosol powder, cream, ointment, powder, solution
Available as Generic? Yes
Drug Class: Topical antifungal

▼ USAGE INFORMATION

WHY IT'S TAKEN
To treat fungal infections of the skin. (Note: Undecylenic acid has generally been replaced by newer and more effective topical antifungal medications; however, your doctor may find it worthwhile to recommend undecylenic acid under certain circumstances—for example, if you have a history of allergic reaction to other antifungal preparations.)

HOW IT WORKS
Undecylenic acid prevents the growth and reproduction of fungus cells.

▼ DOSAGE GUIDELINES

RANGE AND FREQUENCY
Aerosol foam, aerosol powder, ointment, powder, or solution: Apply to the affected area of the skin 2 times a day. The aerosol powder and aerosol spray form of the medicine should be sprayed on the affected area from a distance of 4 to 6 inches. The powder may also be sprayed in socks and shoes. If the powder is used on the feet, sprinkle it between the toes, on the feet, and in shoes and socks. Cream: Apply to the affected area of the skin as often as necessary.

ONSET OF EFFECT
Unknown.

DURATION OF ACTION
Unknown.

DIETARY ADVICE
No special restrictions.

STORAGE
Store in a tightly sealed container away from heat and direct light. Keep aerosol, cream, ointment, and liquid solution forms of undecylenic acid from freezing. Do not puncture, rupture, or incinerate the aerosol container.

MISSED DOSE
Apply a missed dose as soon as you remember. If it is close to the next dose, skip the missed dose and resume your regular dosage schedule. Do not apply a double dose.

STOPPING THE DRUG
Take as recommended for the full treatment period, even if you begin to feel better before the scheduled end of therapy. Discontinuing the drug prematurely may result in an even worse fungal infection later (known as rebound infection). In general, keep using this medication for two weeks after burning, itching, and other symptoms have cleared up.

PROLONGED USE
If your skin problem does not improve or becomes worse after 4 weeks of treatment, consult your doctor.

▼ PRECAUTIONS

Over 60: There is no specific information comparing use of undecylenic acid in older persons with use in patients in other age groups.

Driving and Hazardous Work: No special precautions are necessary.

Alcohol: No special precautions are necessary.

Pregnancy: Undecylenic acid has not been shown to cause birth defects or other problems in humans.

Breast Feeding: Undecylenic acid may pass into breast milk; caution is advised. Consult your doctor for specific advice.

Infants and Children: Not recommended for use on children under age 2.

Special Concerns: Keep this medicine away from the eyes, nose, and mouth. To help prevent reinfection, the powder or spray form of undecylenic acid may be used every day after bathing and careful drying. Do not use on pus-producing sores or on badly broken skin.

OVERDOSE
Symptoms: No specific ones have been reported.

What to Do: An overdose of undecylenic acid is unlikely. However, if someone accidentally ingests the drug, call your doctor, emergency medical services (EMS), or the nearest poison control center.

▼ INTERACTIONS

DRUG INTERACTIONS
Consult your doctor for specific advice if you are taking any other topical prescription or over-the-counter medication that is to be applied to the same area of the skin.

FOOD INTERACTIONS
No known food interactions.

DISEASE INTERACTIONS
Caution is advised when taking undecylenic acid. Consult your doctor if you have any other medical condition that affects the skin.

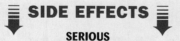

≡ SIDE EFFECTS ≡

SERIOUS
No serious side effects have been reported.

COMMON
No common side effects have been reported.

LESS COMMON
Skin irritation that was not present before use of this medicine. Call your doctor promptly.

VITAMIN A (RETINOL)

BRAND NAMES

Alphalin, Aquasol A, Del-Vi-A, Solaneed, Vi-Dom-A

Available in: Capsules, oral solution, tablets
Available as Generic? Yes
Drug Class: Vitamin

▼ USAGE INFORMATION

WHY IT'S TAKEN
To treat vitamin A deficiency. Most Americans get sufficient amounts of vitamin A from their diet. Most vitamin A is obtained from the conversion of dietary beta-carotene to vitamin A in the intestine. Foods rich in beta-carotene include yellow-orange fruits and vegetables, such as cantaloupe and butternut squash; dark-green leafy vegetables such as spinach and lettuce; liver; and fortified milk and margarine. Supplementation may be necessary with certain medical conditions including long-term chronic illness, liver disorders, intestinal malabsorption associated with chronic diarrhea or pancreatic disease, and surgical removal of the stomach. Vitamin A deficiency can cause night blindness, dry eyes, eye infections, and skin problems.

HOW IT WORKS
Vitamin A plays an essential role in preventing night blindness and in fostering proper growth and maintenance of the skin, bones, and reproductive organs.

▼ DOSAGE GUIDELINES

RANGE AND FREQUENCY
For severe vitamin A deficiency: 100,000 International Units (IU) daily for 3 days, followed by 25,000 to 50,000 IU daily for 2 weeks, then 10,000 to 20,000 IU daily for 2 months. To prevent vitamin deficiency (recommended daily allowance)—Adults: 3,330 IU daily for men, 2,665 IU daily for women. Children ages 7 to 10: 2,330 IU daily. Children ages 4 to 6: 1,665 IU daily. Children ages 1 to 3: 1,330 IU daily. Infants: 1,250 IU daily.

ONSET OF EFFECT
Unknown.

DURATION OF ACTION
Unknown.

DIETARY ADVICE
Absorption of vitamin A requires some fat in the diet.

STORAGE
Store in a tightly sealed container away from heat, moisture, and direct light.

MISSED DOSE
Take it as soon as you remember you should.

STOPPING THE DRUG
If you are taking vitamin A because of a deficiency, use it as directed for the full treatment period.

PROLONGED USE
Prolonged use of high doses may cause serious toxicity (see Overdose).

▼ PRECAUTIONS

Over 60: Adverse reactions associated with high-dose, long-term use may be more likely and more severe in older patients.

Driving and Hazardous Work: The use of recommended doses of vitamin A should not impair your ability to perform such tasks safely.

Alcohol: No special precautions are necessary.

Pregnancy: An adequate vitamin A intake is essential during pregnancy. However, a vitamin A overdose (more than 6,000 IU daily) can cause birth defects or slow or reduce growth in the fetus.

Breast Feeding: Vitamin A passes into breast milk; caution is advised. Ingesting too much vitamin A during breast feeding can be harmful to the nursing infant.

Infants and Children: Children are more sensitive to side effects from high doses of vitamin A.

Special Concerns: Vitamin A can be highly toxic (see Overdose) when taken in high doses. Take only as directed.

OVERDOSE
Symptoms: Acute overdose: Bleeding from gums, sore mouth, confusion or unusual excitement, diarrhea, drowsiness or dizziness, double vision, severe headache, irritability, peeling skin, especially on lips and palms, severe vomiting. Chronic overdose (with prolonged overuse): Drying or cracking of skin or lips, bone or joint pain, fever, general feeling of discomfort, increased sensitivity of skin to sunlight, increased urination, loss of appetite, hair loss, stomach pain, unusual fatigue, yellow-orange patches on soles of feet, palms of hands, or skin around the nose and lips.

What to Do: For an acute overdose, call your doctor, emergency medical services (EMS), or the nearest poison control center immediately. For symptoms of chronic overdose, be sure to talk to your doctor.

▼ INTERACTIONS

DRUG INTERACTIONS
Consult your doctor for specific advice if you are taking etretinate or isotretinoin.

FOOD INTERACTIONS
No known food interactions.

DISEASE INTERACTIONS
Consult your doctor before taking vitamin A if you have a history of alcohol abuse, liver disease, or kidney disease.

≡ SIDE EFFECTS ≡

SERIOUS
No serious side effects occur with recommended doses of vitamin A (see Overdose).

COMMON
No common side effects occur with recommended doses of vitamin A.

LESS COMMON
No less-common side effects occur with recommended doses of vitamin A.

VITAMIN B1 (THIAMINE)

Thiamilate

Available in: Tablets
Available as Generic? Yes
Drug Class: Vitamin

▼ USAGE INFORMATION

WHY IT'S TAKEN
To prevent and treat a vitamin B1 deficiency. Vitamin B1 deficiency can lead to either beriberi, which affects many body tissues, including the heart and nervous system (symptoms include constipation, loss of appetite, pain or tingling in arms and legs, emaciation, paralysis, heart failure, and mental deficits), or a severe brain disorder known as Wernicke's encephalopathy.

HOW IT WORKS
Thiamine is one of the B-complex vitamins, which are essential for normal metabolism and for the health and proper functioning of the cardiovascular and nervous systems. Thiamine is required for the formation of a factor needed for the function of enzymes involved in the metabolism of carbohydrates.

▼ DOSAGE GUIDELINES

RANGE AND FREQUENCY
Recommended daily allowance—Infants, birth to 3 years: 0.4 mg per day.

Children ages 4 to 6: 0.9 mg. Children ages 7 to 10: 1 mg. Males ages 11 to 14: 1.3 mg. Males ages 15 to 50: 1.5 mg. Males ages 51 and over: 1.2 mg. Women ages 11 to 50: 1.1 mg. Women ages 51 and over: 1 mg. Breast-feeding women: 1.6 mg. Pregnant women: 1.5 mg. To treat beriberi—Adults and teenagers: 5 to 10 mg, 3 times a day. Children: 10 mg a day.

ONSET OF EFFECT
Unknown.

DURATION OF ACTION
Unknown.

DIETARY ADVICE
Take it with or between meals.

STORAGE
Store in a tightly sealed container away from moisture, heat, and direct light.

MISSED DOSE
Take it as soon as you realize you forgot a dose.

STOPPING THE DRUG
If thiamine is being taken to treat beriberi, a serious medical condition, the decision to stop taking the drug should be made by your doctor.

▼ SIDE EFFECTS

▼ SERIOUS ▼
There are no serious side effects associated with the use of thiamine (except in very rare cases pertaining to high doses administered by injection, which occur exclusively in a hospital setting).

COMMON
No common side effects have been reported.

LESS COMMON
No less-common side effects have been reported.

PROLONGED USE
No problems are expected.

▼ PRECAUTIONS

Over 60: No problems have been reported in older persons, who are more likely to have low blood levels of thiamine and thus require a dietary supplement.

Driving and Hazardous Work: No special precautions are necessary.

Alcohol: No special precautions are necessary.

Pregnancy: A vitamin supplement containing thiamine may be recommended, but taking large amounts of a supplement during pregnancy may be harmful to the mother or fetus. Consult your doctor for advice.

Breast Feeding: Taking large amounts of a dietary supplement while breast feeding may be harmful to the infant. Consult your doctor for specific advice. If thiamine deficiency occurs during breast feeding, a doctor should treat both the mother and the nursing infant.

Infants and Children: No problems have been reported in infants and children with the intake of recommended daily allowances.

Special Concerns: Develop good nutritional habits to avoid a vitamin B1 deficiency. Thiamine-rich foods include pork, organ meats, green leafy vegetables, legumes, sweet corn, corn meal, egg yolks, brown rice, yeast, whole grains, berries, and nuts. Supplements of more than 15 mg taken 3 times a day are poorly absorbed from the intestine.

OVERDOSE
Symptoms: There have been no cases of thiamine overdose reported.

What to Do: Emergency instructions not applicable.

▼ INTERACTIONS

DRUG INTERACTIONS
Consult your doctor for specific advice if you are taking any other prescription or OTC medication.

FOOD INTERACTIONS
No known food interactions.

DISEASE INTERACTIONS
Thiamine deficiency is most likely to occur in people on extremely low-calorie diets or persons who suffer from a gastrointestinal disease (leading to chronic malabsorption), cirrhosis, or alcoholism. A clinically significant deficiency can occur after only a few weeks of a diet with little or no thiamine.

VITAMIN B2 (RIBOFLAVIN)

Available in: Tablets, sugar-free tablets
Available as Generic? Yes
Drug Class: Dietary supplement

▼ USAGE INFORMATION

WHY IT'S TAKEN
To treat vitamin B2 deficiency. Riboflavin must be included in the nutrients administered to patients receiving all their nutrition intravenously. A riboflavin deficiency may have symptoms that include sensitivity of eyes to light; itching and burning eyes; itching and peeling skin on the nose and scrotum; and sores at the corners of the mouth and on the tongue. Riboflavin requirements may be increased in people suffering from severe burns, chronic diarrhea, cirrhosis of the liver, alcoholism, cancer, or in those who have undergone surgical removal of the stomach.

HOW IT WORKS
Riboflavin is one of the B-complex vitamins, which are essential for normal metabolism and for the health and function of the cardiovascular and nervous systems. Specifically, body cells convert riboflavin into two products essential to the activity of enzymes that break down carbohydrates, proteins, and fats, and that enable oxygen to be used by the body's cells.

▼ DOSAGE GUIDELINES

RANGE AND FREQUENCY
Recommended intakes—Adult and teenage males: 1.4 to 1.8 mg daily. Adult and teenage females: 1.2 to 1.3 mg daily. Children ages 7 to 10: 1.2 mg daily. Children ages 4 to 6: 1.1 mg daily. Infants from birth to 3: 0.4 to 0.8 mg daily. Pregnant women: 1.6 mg daily. Breast-feeding women: 1.7 to 1.8 mg daily. Sufficient vitamin B2 is usually provided by adequate diets.

ONSET OF EFFECT
Unknown.

DURATION OF ACTION
Unknown.

DIETARY ADVICE
Avoid alcohol; it reduces the absorption of riboflavin from the intestine.

STORAGE
Store in a tightly sealed container away from moisture, heat, and direct light.

MISSED DOSE
Take it as soon as you remember. No problems are expected as a result of missing a dose.

STOPPING THE DRUG
If your doctor has recommended riboflavin for a vitamin deficiency, take it as prescribed for the full treatment period.

PROLONGED USE
No special problems are expected.

▼ PRECAUTIONS

Over 60: No special problems are expected.

Driving and Hazardous Work: No special precautions are necessary.

Alcohol: Alcohol may reduce the absorption of vitamin B2 from the intestine.

Pregnancy: No known problems. Riboflavin requirements are increased slightly during pregnancy.

Breast Feeding: Recommended intake of riboflavin and other vitamins is increased during breast feeding. Taking excessive amounts while breast feeding may be harmful to the nursing baby. Consult your doctor for specific advice.

Infants and Children: No problems are expected.

Special Concerns: Riboflavin supplements may cause a harmless yellow discoloration of the urine. Severe weight-reducing diets may reduce riboflavin intake below recommended amounts, and require supplementation or increased intake of riboflavin-rich foods like eggs, organ meats, whole-grain cereals and breads, green leafy vegetables, mushrooms, avocados, legumes (such as kidney beans), cashews, chestnuts, milk, and cheeses.

OVERDOSE
Symptoms: No specific ones have been reported.

What to Do: Emergency instructions not applicable.

▼ INTERACTIONS

DRUG INTERACTIONS
Consult your doctor for advice about dietary supplements if you are taking propantheline, phenothiazines, tricyclic antidepressants, or probenecid.

FOOD INTERACTIONS
None expected.

DISEASE INTERACTIONS
None expected.

≡ SIDE EFFECTS ≡

SERIOUS
No serious side effects have been reported.

COMMON
Urine may appear bright yellow when riboflavin is taken in high doses.

LESS COMMON
No less-common side effects have been reported.

VITAMIN B3 (NIACIN)

BRAND NAMES

Niacin-Time, Niacinol, Niaspan, Nicobid, Nicolar, Slo-niacin

Available in: Tablets, extended-release tablets
Available as Generic? Yes
Drug Class: Dietary supplement; antilipidemic (lipid-lowering) agent

▼ USAGE INFORMATION

WHY IT'S TAKEN
As a dietary supplement: To prevent or treat niacin deficiency (pellagra). Symptoms include dermatitis, diarrhea, and dementia. (Healthy people eating a well-rounded diet do not develop niacin deficiency.) As an antilipidemic: Large doses of niacin are used to lower total and LDL cholesterol and triglyceride levels. It is the most effective drug currently available to increase HDL cholesterol levels.

HOW IT WORKS
Niacin is required for the proper action of enzymes involved in energy metabolism. It lowers blood lipids by partially blocking the release of fatty acids from adipose (fat) tissue and reducing the liver's production of the triglyceride-carrying lipoprotein, very-low- density lipoprotein (VLDL).

▼ DOSAGE GUIDELINES

RANGE AND FREQUENCY
Tablets—Recommended daily allowances for niacin are 5 to 15 mg a day for children; 15 to 20 mg a day for adolescent and adult men; and 13 to 15 mg a day for adolescent and adult women. To treat pellagra: 250 to 500 mg a day. As an antilipidemic: 500 to 4,500 mg a day in divided doses with meals. Extended-release tablets—As an antilipidemic: All doses are taken once a day at bedtime following a low-fat snack. Week 1: 375 mg. Week 2: 500 mg. Week 3: 750 mg. Weeks 4 to 7: 1,000 mg. After week 7, your doctor will evaluate your response to your dose.

ONSET OF EFFECT
2 to 4 weeks.

DURATION OF ACTION
As long as it is taken.

DIETARY ADVICE
A well-balanced diet will prevent niacin deficiency.

STORAGE
Avoid heat and direct light.

MISSED DOSE
Skip the missed dose and resume you regular dosage schedule. Do not double the next dose.

STOPPING THE DRUG
If you take this vitamin as an antilipidemic, do not stop unless so instructed by your doctor. Once niacin is stopped, lipids will increase to pretreatment levels.

PROLONGED USE
Side effects are more likely with prolonged use.

▼ PRECAUTIONS

Over 60: Possible increase in side effects and risk of developing diabetes.

Driving and Hazardous Work: No special precautions are necessary.

Alcohol: Niacin deficiency is more common in alcoholics because of their poor diets. Alcohol can increase blood triglycerides in people with blood lipid abnormalities. Alcohol also increases the risk of flushing reactions.

Pregnancy: Pregnancy increases a woman's dietary niacin needs to 17 to 20 mg a day. If this vitamin is taken as an antilipidemic, however, niacin therapy should be discontinued unless the doctor believes benefits clearly outweigh possible risks.

Breast Feeding: Breast feeding increases dietary niacin needs to 20 mg a day. There is no evidence of danger to the infant from niacin as an antilipidemic, but your doctor should reconsider whether continued therapy is absolutely necessary.

Infants and Children: Safety has not been established for treatment of lipid problems.

Special Concerns: Periodic tests to assess liver function, blood glucose, and uric acid levels are needed.

OVERDOSE
Symptoms: Flushing, abdominal pain, nausea, vomiting.

What to Do: Call your doctor.

▼ INTERACTIONS

DRUG INTERACTIONS
Niacin combined with HMG-CoA reductase inhibitors (lipid-lowering drugs known as statins) can cause myositis (muscle inflammation) with muscle pain and tenderness. Severe myositis can damage kidneys and lead to kidney failure. The drugs must be stopped immediately if symptoms of myositis occur.

FOOD INTERACTIONS
Flushing may be worse when niacin is taken with hot foods or drinks.

DISEASE INTERACTIONS
Niacin should not be used by those with a history of gout or peptic ulcer. It should be used with caution by people with diabetes, borderline high glucose levels, or any evidence of liver abnormalities.

☰ SIDE EFFECTS ☰

▼ SERIOUS ▼
Liver toxicity leading to jaundice (yellow discoloration of skin and eyes) and fatigue (more common with slow-release forms of niacin); gastrointestinal irritation causing nausea, vomiting, and abdominal pain; peptic ulcer; increased uric acid levels leading to gout attacks; elevated blood glucose levels.

COMMON
Itching, flushing, sweating, and dizziness, often within 20 to 40 minutes after taking niacin. These symptoms can usually be reduced or eliminated by taking an aspirin 30 minutes before the niacin. They tend to diminish or disappear with prolonged use. Slow-release forms reduce these side effects. Nausea and vomiting may also occur.

LESS COMMON
Dry skin, headaches, eye problems.

VITAMIN B6 (PYRIDOXINE)

BRAND NAMES
Beesix, Doxine, Nestrex, Pyri, Rodex, Vitabee 6

Available in: Tablets
Available as Generic? Yes
Drug Class: Dietary supplement

▼ USAGE INFORMATION

WHY IT'S TAKEN
To treat or prevent vitamin B6 deficiency, which can cause anemia, dermatitis, nervous system problems, and painful cracking at the outer sides of the mouth. Deficiency does not occur in healthy people eating a well-balanced diet. However, several genetic abnormalities may lead to a higher vitamin B6 requirement than can be obtained from the diet. Supplements may also be necessary in people with alcoholism, an overactive thyroid, or intestinal diseases associated with nutritional malabsorption.

HOW IT WORKS
Vitamin B6 is used to manufacture a substance required for the proper action of enzymes involved in the metabolism of carbohydrates, fats, and proteins.

▼ DOSAGE GUIDELINES

RANGE AND FREQUENCY
Recommended daily allowances for vitamin B6 are 0.3 to 1 mg from birth to age 3; 1.1 mg from age 4 to 7; 1.4 mg from age 7 to 10; 1.7 to 2 mg in adolescent and adult males; and 1.4 to 1.6 mg in adolescent and adult females. For vitamin B6 deficiency or an inherited abnormality causing increased vitamin B6 requirements, consult your doctor.

ONSET OF EFFECT
Unknown.

DURATION OF ACTION
As long as the vitamin is taken.

DIETARY ADVICE
Eat a well-balanced diet. Foods rich in vitamin B6 include egg yolks, meats, bananas, and whole grain cereals.

STORAGE
Store in a cool, dry place.

MISSED DOSE
Take the next regularly scheduled dose.

STOPPING THE DRUG
If the vitamin was prescribed for a deficiency, consult your doctor before stopping.

PROLONGED USE
No problems are expected with recommended doses of vitamin B6.

▼ PRECAUTIONS

Over 60: No special problems are to be expected with recommended doses.

Driving and Hazardous Work: No special precautions are necessary.

Alcohol: Alcoholism can lead to a vitamin B6 deficiency. Conversely, those who are being treated for vitamin B6 deficiency should abstain from alcohol.

Pregnancy: Vitamin B6 requirements increase during pregnancy to 2.2 mg per day. Very large doses may cause vitamin B6 dependency in the newborn child.

Breast Feeding: Vitamin B6 requirements increase during breast feeding to 2.1 mg per day.

Infants and Children: No problems are expected with recommended doses.

OVERDOSE
Symptoms: Overdose is extremely rare. Two cases that caused central nervous system toxicity (see Serious Side Effects) have been reported.

What to Do: Although an overdose is highly unlikely to occur, call your doctor right away if you have any reason to suspect that one has occurred.

▼ INTERACTIONS

DRUG INTERACTIONS
Vitamin B6 is used in the treatment of toxicity from the drugs cycloserine and isoniazid. Other drugs that may increase the daily requirement for vitamin B6 include ethionamide, hydralazine, penicillamine, immunosuppressants, and estrogen.

FOOD INTERACTIONS
No food interactions have been reported.

DISEASE INTERACTIONS
No disease interactions have been reported.

≡ SIDE EFFECTS ≡

SERIOUS
When taken for several months, high doses of vitamin B6 (2 to 6 grams daily) may cause reversible nerve damage; symptoms include numbness, tingling, or prickling in the feet, loss of manual dexterity, and unsteady gait.

COMMON
No common side effects are associated with recommended doses.

LESS COMMON
No less-common side effects are associated with recommended doses.

VITAMIN B12 (CYANOCOBALAMIN)

Available in: Tablets, extended-release tablets
Available as Generic? Yes
Drug Class: Dietary supplement

▼ USAGE INFORMATION

WHY IT'S TAKEN
Cyanocobalamin is a synthetic form of vitamin B12, used to correct a vitamin B12 deficiency and to remedy the associated medical conditions (anemia and nerve damage) that may result from such a deficiency. A B12 deficiency can occur for a number of reasons, including a diet lacking in animal protein, pernicious anemia, intestinal malabsorption, surgical removal of portions of the stomach or small intestine, the effects of certain drugs (including colchicine, neomycin, and PAS), or because an individual is unable to keep up with an increase in the daily requirements of the vitamin (as occurs during pregnancy or during periods of great physical stress).

HOW IT WORKS
Vitamin B12 is essential for the proper production of blood platelets and red and white blood cells, the manufacture of vital substances needed for cell function, and the metabolism of nutrients necessary for cell growth.

▼ DOSAGE GUIDELINES

RANGE AND FREQUENCY
Recommended daily allowances (RDA)—Adults and teenagers: 2 micrograms (mcg). Pregnant or nursing women: 2.2 mcg. Children ages 7 to 10: 1.4 mcg. Children ages 4 to 6: 1 mcg. From birth to 3 years of age: 0.3 to 0.7 mcg. (Extended-release tablets are not recommended for children.) To treat a severe vitamin B12 deficiency—The dose will be determined by your doctor based on individual criteria.

ONSET OF EFFECT
Immediate.

DURATION OF ACTION
For as long as the supplement is taken.

DIETARY ADVICE
Eat a healthy, well-balanced diet. Foods rich in vitamin B12 include animal protein, clams and oysters, liver, fish, milk, and egg yolks.

STORAGE
Store in a tightly sealed container away from moisture, heat, and direct light.

MISSED DOSE
Take the next regularly scheduled dose.

STOPPING THE DRUG
If the vitamin was prescribed for a deficiency, consult your doctor before stopping.

PROLONGED USE
Therapy may require weeks or months. For certain conditions, lifelong therapy is sometimes necessary. No problems are expected with prolonged use, however, when the vitamin is taken as directed.

▼ PRECAUTIONS

Over 60: No special problems are expected with recommended doses.

Driving and Hazardous Work: No special precautions are necessary.

Alcohol: Alcoholism can lead to pancreatic insufficiency and vitamin B12 malabsorption.

Pregnancy: Vitamin B12 requirements increase during pregnancy to 2.2 mcg daily.

Breast Feeding: Vitamin B12 requirements increase during breast feeding to 2.2 mcg per day.

Infants and Children: No problems are expected with recommended doses.

Special Concerns: Vitamin B12 deficiency is highly unlikely to occur in healthy people who are able to consume a normal, balanced diet. However, nutritional supplements should be considered for those who are ill or weakened by radiation therapy, chemotherapy, or any other condition that interferes with normal food and fluid intake. Vitamin supplements are not a substitute for a healthy, balanced diet.

OVERDOSE
Symptoms: Overdose is extremely rare.

What to Do: Although an overdose is highly unlikely, call your doctor right away if you have any reason to suspect that one has occurred.

▼ INTERACTIONS

DRUG INTERACTIONS
Consult your doctor for specific advice if you are taking analgesics, antibiotics, folic acid, colchicine, or other vitamin supplements.

FOOD INTERACTIONS
No known food interactions.

DISEASE INTERACTIONS
Consult your doctor about dietary supplements if you have Leber's disease (a very rare eye disease).

≡ SIDE EFFECTS ≡

SERIOUS
Breathing difficulty, fever, hives, rash, swelling of face, mouth, lips, throat, or tongue. These may be signs of a rare but potentially serious allergic reaction. Seek medical assistance immediately.

COMMON
No common side effects have been reported with recommended doses.

LESS COMMON
Mild allergic reaction, diarrhea, itching.

VITAMIN C (ASCORBIC ACID)

Available in: Tablets, capsules
Available as Generic? Yes
Drug Class: Dietary supplement

▼ USAGE INFORMATION

WHY IT'S TAKEN
To prevent or treat vitamin C deficiency, or scurvy, a disorder characterized by bleeding into the skin, swollen and bleeding gums, poor wound healing, muscle weakness, and fatigue. Deficiency does not occur in healthy people eating a well-balanced diet. Vitamin C requirements may be increased in those with AIDS, alcoholism, overactive thyroid, chronic infection, and intestinal diseases associated with nutritional malabsorption.

HOW IT WORKS
Vitamin C is required for the body's synthesis of collagen (tissue that constitutes the tendons, ligaments, and other inelastic fibers), for the metabolism of a variety of body substances, and to maintain structural and functional integrity of cell walls and small blood vessels.

▼ DOSAGE GUIDELINES

RANGE AND FREQUENCY
Recommended daily allowances for vitamin C are as follows: 30 to 40 mg from birth to 3 years of age; 45 mg from age 4 to 10; 50 to 60 mg in adolescents and adults; 100 mg in smokers.

ONSET OF EFFECT
Unknown.

DURATION OF ACTION
As long as it is taken.

DIETARY ADVICE
Eat a well-balanced diet to avoid vitamin C deficiency. Foods rich in vitamin C include citrus fruits and juices, strawberries, green vegetables, and tomatoes.

STORAGE
Store in tightly sealed container away from moisture, heat, and direct light.

MISSED DOSE
No problems are expected if a dose is forgotten. Take the next dose at the regularly scheduled time and do not double the next dose.

STOPPING THE DRUG
If vitamin C is taken for a deficiency or because of a disorder associated with nutritional requirements for the vitamin, consult your doctor before stopping your use.

PROLONGED USE
No problems are expected with prolonged use.

▼ PRECAUTIONS

Over 60: No special problems are expected.

Driving and Hazardous Work: No special precautions are necessary.

Alcohol: Alcoholism may lead to vitamin C deficiency.

Pregnancy: Vitamin C requirements increase during pregnancy to 70 mg per day. Very large doses during pregnancy may harm the fetus.

Breast Feeding: Vitamin C requirements increase during breast feeding to 90 to 95 mg per day. Vitamin C does enter breast milk, but so far no problems have been reported from taking the recommended amounts of it.

Infants and Children: No problems are associated with recommended doses.

Special Concerns: Use of large doses of vitamin C is commonplace for the prevention of colds, cancer, and other disorders. Studies have shown that blood levels of the vitamin do not increase further when vitamin C doses exceed 250 to 500 mg per day. High doses of vitamin C may cause kidney stones in people with a prior history of the disorder or those with kidney disease being treated with hemodialysis.

OVERDOSE
Symptoms: No specific ones have been reported.

What to Do: Emergency instructions not applicable.

▼ INTERACTIONS

DRUG INTERACTIONS
None reported with recommended doses.

FOOD INTERACTIONS
No known food interactions. However, it is worth noting that vitamin C can improve the body's absorption of iron, specifically nonheme iron (the type of iron found in foods derived from plant sources).

DISEASE INTERACTIONS
None reported.

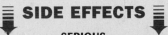

≡ SIDE EFFECTS ≡

SERIOUS
Occasionally, kidney stones may develop (especially with doses greater than 1 g per day over a prolonged period of time), causing back, side, or flank pain.

COMMON
No common side effects are associated with recommended doses.

LESS COMMON
High doses may cause diarrhea, flushing and redness of the skin, nausea and vomiting, or headache.

VITAMIN D

BRAND NAME

Drisdol

Available in: Capsules, oral solution, tablets
Available as Generic? Yes
Drug Class: Dietary supplement

▼ USAGE INFORMATION

WHY IT'S TAKEN
Vitamin D is necessary for good health, and especially to maintain strong, healthy bones. It is derived from dietary sources, plus the body manufactures its own vitamin D upon exposure to sunlight. Vitamin D deficiency is thus rare among Americans, but some people–notably, individuals who are bedridden, have poor or highly restricted (vegan or macrobiotic) diets, or who cannot get adequate nutrition due to intestinal malabsorption–require supplementation. In addition, dietary supplements may be recommended for people with chronically low blood levels of calcium, and for alcoholics, dark-skinned people (who manufacture smaller amounts of vitamin D on their own), pregnant women, and nursing infants who get inadequate exposure to sunlight. Vitamin D supplements are also often recommended to increase calcium absorption and prevent osteoporosis in postmenopausal women.

HOW IT WORKS
Vitamin D promotes the absorption of calcium from the intestine and the utilization of calcium and phosphorus in the body. This ensures that levels of these minerals are high enough to support the constant breakdown and rebuilding of bone tissue, and to supply cells with the calcium needed to perform essential functions. Some tablets contain both vitamin D and calcium.

▼ DOSAGE GUIDELINES

RANGE AND FREQUENCY
Recommended daily allowances–Adults and teens: 200 to 400 international units (IU). Infants and children up to age 12: 300 to 400 IU. Pregnant or breast-feeding women: 400 IU. Vitamin D supplementation for deficiency, osteoporosis prevention or other medical condition– Same as above or higher, as determined by your doctor.

ONSET OF EFFECT
Within 12 to 24 hours; maximum effect: 10 to 14 days.

DURATION OF ACTION
As long as vitamin is taken.

DIETARY ADVICE
The best sources of vitamin D are fish and milk fortified with vitamin D.

STORAGE
Store in a tightly sealed container away from heat and direct light.

MISSED DOSE
When vitamin D is used as a dietary supplement, no problems are expected if you miss a dose. When it is prescribed to treat a specific medical condition, take the missed dose as soon as you remember. If it is near the time for the next dose, skip the missed dose and resume your regular dosage schedule. Do not double the next dose.

STOPPING THE DRUG
If you are taking the supplement on your doctor's advice, do not stop without first consulting him or her.

PROLONGED USE
Your doctor will take periodic blood tests to check levels of calcium and phosphorus if you are taking vitamin D for the treatment of low blood calcium levels.

▼ PRECAUTIONS

Over 60: No special problems are expected.

Driving and Hazardous Work: No special precautions.

Alcohol: No special warnings.

Pregnancy: Daily requirements for vitamin D increase during pregnancy.

Breast Feeding: Trace amounts pass into breast milk; however, no problems have been reported. Vitamin D intake should in fact be increased while nursing.

Infants and Children: Infants who get little exposure to the sun and are totally breast-fed, especially those with dark-skinned mothers, may require vitamin D supplementation. Problems have not been reported with recommended amounts; however, prolonged excess doses may stunt a child's growth.

OVERDOSE
Symptoms: Early symptoms: Constipation (especially in children), diarrhea, dry mouth, increased thirst and frequency of urination, persistent headache, loss of appetite, metallic taste, nausea and vomiting, unusual fatigue. Advanced symptoms: Bone and muscle pain, irregular heartbeat, persistent itching, extreme drowsiness, mental changes. Severe vitamin D toxicity may be fatal.

What to Do: See your doctor at once.

▼ INTERACTIONS

DRUG INTERACTIONS
Consult your doctor for specific advice if you are taking calcium-containing preparations, magnesium-containing antacids, or thiazide diuretics.

FOOD INTERACTIONS
No known food interactions.

DISEASE INTERACTIONS
Consult your doctor before taking vitamin D if you have high blood levels of calcium (hypercalcemia), or a history of heart or blood vessel disease, pancreatitis, or impaired kidney function.

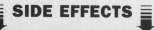

≡ SIDE EFFECTS ≡
▼ **SERIOUS** ▼
Serious side effects are associated with excessively high doses (see Overdose).

COMMON
No side effects are expected with recommended doses.

LESS COMMON
No side effects are expected with recommended doses.

VITAMIN E (TOCOPHEROL)

Available in: Capsules
Available as Generic? Yes
Drug Class: Dietary supplement

▼ USAGE INFORMATION

WHY IT'S TAKEN
For the prevention and treatment of vitamin E deficiency. Vitamin E deficiency is extremely rare and does not occur in healthy individuals eating a well-balanced diet. However, a deficiency of vitamin E can result from any disorder that causes poor absorption of fat from the intestine. Vitamin E is an antioxidant that is often prescribed to prevent the oxidation of low-density lipoprotein in an effort to prevent atherosclerosis (buildup of fatty plaques within the arteries), the underlying cause of coronary heart disease. The value of vitamin E supplements for this purpose is unproven.

HOW IT WORKS
Although considered an essential vitamin, the exact function of vitamin E remains unknown. It does help to prevent oxidation of the fatty acids present in the membranes of all cells (that is, it has antioxidant properties).

▼ DOSAGE GUIDELINES

RANGE AND FREQUENCY
Daily vitamin E requirements are small, ranging from 5 international units (IU) at birth to 20 IU in breast-feeding women. Large doses (100 IU) are given when deficiency results from intestinal malabsorption. The usual doses prescribed for protection against coronary heart disease range from 400 to 800 IU per day.

ONSET OF EFFECT
Unknown.

DURATION OF ACTION
Unknown.

DIETARY ADVICE
Eat a well-balanced diet. Foods rich in vitamin E include vegetable oils, whole grains, and leafy green vegetables. Cooking and storage may cause significant losses of vitamin E.

STORAGE
Store in a tightly sealed container away from moisture, heat, and direct light.

MISSED DOSE
No problems are expected. Take the next dose at the regularly scheduled time and do not double the next dose.

STOPPING THE DRUG
If prescribed for a deficiency, do not stop taking vitamin E without consulting your doctor first. There is no evidence that stopping vitamin E when it is taken to prevent coronary heart disease is harmful.

PROLONGED USE
No problems are associated with prolonged use.

▼ PRECAUTIONS

Over 60: No problems are expected with vitamin E at recommended doses.

Driving and Hazardous Work: No special precautions are necessary.

Alcohol: No special precautions are necessary.

Pregnancy: No problems are expected with vitamin E at recommended doses.

Breast Feeding: Vitamin E enters breast milk, but no problems have been reported with recommended doses.

Infants and Children: No problems have been documented with vitamin E at recommended doses.

OVERDOSE
Symptoms: There have been no reported cases of vitamin E overdose.

What to Do: Emergency instructions not applicable.

▼ INTERACTIONS

DRUG INTERACTIONS
Consumption of large doses of vitamin E in combination with anticoagulants (such as warfarin) might lead to uncontrolled bleeding.

FOOD INTERACTIONS
Absorption of vitamin E from the intestine requires the consumption of some dietary fat.

DISEASE INTERACTIONS
No disease interactions have been reported.

≣ SIDE EFFECTS ≣

SERIOUS
No serious side effects are associated with recommended doses.

COMMON
No common side effects are associated with recommended doses.

LESS COMMON
Large doses (greater than 400 IU per day) have been associated with diarrhea, nausea, headache, blurred vision, dizziness, and fatigue. Doses greater than 800 IU per day have been reported to increase the danger of bleeding, especially in people deficient in vitamin K.

YOHIMBINE

BRAND NAMES

Actibine, Aphrodyne, Baron-X, Dayton Himbin, Prohim, Thybine, Yocon, Yohimar, Yohimex, Yoman, Yovital

Available in: Tablets
Available as Generic? Yes
Drug Class: Alpha-adrenergic blocking agent

▼ USAGE INFORMATION

WHY IT'S TAKEN
To aid in the treatment of male erectile dysfunction (impotence).

HOW IT WORKS
The exact way that yohimbine works has not been determined. It is believed to block certain chemical receptors that cause constriction of blood vessels. In doing so, yohimbine theoretically improves blood flow into (and inhibits blood flow out of) the spongy columns of tissue in the penis involved in the mechanics of erection. Yohimbine may also have a mild stimulant effect and may promote the release of brain chemicals that control mood, relaxation, and sex drive, among other functions.

▼ DOSAGE GUIDELINES

RANGE AND FREQUENCY
Adult males: 5.4 mg, 3 times a day.

ONSET OF EFFECT
Occurs within 2 to 3 weeks in most cases.

DURATION OF ACTION
Unknown.

DIETARY ADVICE
No special restrictions.

STORAGE
Store in a tightly sealed container away from moisture, heat, and direct light. Do not refrigerate medication or allow it to freeze.

MISSED DOSE
Take it as soon as you remember. If it is near the time for the next dose, skip the missed dose and resume your regular dosage schedule. Do not double the next dose.

STOPPING THE DRUG
If your doctor has recommended yohimbine, consult him or her before stopping.

PROLONGED USE
See your doctor regularly for tests and examinations if you take this drug for a prolonged period of time.

▼ PRECAUTIONS

Over 60: No special problems are expected.

Driving and Hazardous Work: Do not drive or engage in hazardous work until you determine how the medicine affects you.

Alcohol: There are no special restrictions; however, excess alcohol consumption may impair sexual function.

Pregnancy: Yohimbine is generally not prescribed for women and should not be used during pregnancy.

Breast Feeding: Not applicable to female patients.

Infants and Children: Not applicable to children.

Special Concerns: This drug should be used only by men who have been diagnosed with and are being medically treated for erectile dysfunction.

OVERDOSE
Symptoms: Agitation, restlessness, dizziness, and rapid or irregular heartbeat.

What to Do: An overdose with yohimbine is unlikely. However, if someone takes a much larger dose than prescribed, call your doctor, emergency medical services (EMS), or the nearest poison control center.

▼ INTERACTIONS

DRUG INTERACTIONS
Consult your doctor for specific advice if you are taking antidepressants (especially MAO inhibitors) or any other mood-modifying medications, including selective serotonin reuptake inhibitors (SSRIs), such as fluoxetine. Before you take yohimbine, tell your doctor if you are taking any other prescription or OTC drugs, especially cold remedies or weight-loss aids.

FOOD INTERACTIONS
Since yohimbine is a mild MAO inhibitor, it should not be taken with any food or drink containing tyramines, including cheese, chocolate, beer, aged meats, and nuts, and particularly not with the amino acids tyrosine or phenylalanine. The combination may cause a dangerous rise in blood pressure.

DISEASE INTERACTIONS
Caution is advised when taking yohimbine. Consult your doctor if you have a history of angina pectoris, mental depression or any other psychiatric illness, heart disease, high blood pressure, or impaired kidney function. Use of yohimbine may cause complications in patients with liver disease, since this organ works to remove the medication from the body.

≡ SIDE EFFECTS ≡

▼ SERIOUS ▼
Rapid heartbeat; increased blood pressure, possibly causing symptoms such as persistent headaches or ringing in the ears. Call your doctor immediately.

COMMON
No common side effects have been reported.

LESS COMMON
Headache, dizziness, irritability, nervousness, restlessness, flushing of skin, shakiness, increased sweating.

ZINC OXIDE

BRAND NAMES

Ken Tox

Available in: Cream, ointment
Available as Generic? Yes
Drug Class: Sunscreen

▼ USAGE INFORMATION

WHY IT'S TAKEN
To prevent sunburn.

HOW IT WORKS
Zinc oxide blocks ultraviolet radiation in sunlight from reaching the skin.

▼ DOSAGE GUIDELINES

RANGE AND FREQUENCY
Apply as needed before exposure to sunlight. A sunscreen should be applied uniformly to all exposed skin surfaces, including the lips.

ONSET OF EFFECT
Immediate.

DURATION OF ACTION
Keeps working until removed or worn off from perspiration or swimming.

DIETARY ADVICE
Zinc oxide can be used without regard to diet.

STORAGE
Store in a tightly sealed container away from heat and direct light.

MISSED DOSE
If you forget to apply zinc oxide before exposure to sunlight, apply as soon as you think of it.

STOPPING THE DRUG
No special warnings.

PROLONGED USE
No problems are expected.

▼ PRECAUTIONS

Over 60: Studies suggest that frequent use of sunscreens like zinc oxide may increase the risk of vitamin D deficiency, which may promote osteoporosis or bone fractures later in life. Oral vitamin D supplements and consumption of foods rich in vitamin D may be recommended.

Driving and Hazardous Work: The use of zinc oxide should not impair your ability to perform such tasks safely.

Alcohol: No special precautions are necessary.

Pregnancy: No problems have been reported.

Breast Feeding: No problems have been reported.

Infants and Children: Zinc oxide should not be used on children (especially infants under 6 months of age) who have shown signs of allergic skin reaction (hypersensitivity). Otherwise, it is safe for use in children. To prevent accidental ingestion, do not allow small children to apply sunscreens themselves. In general, children should be kept out of the sun during peak daylight hours (from 10 am to 2 pm) and physically protected from direct sun exposure with clothing and other physical barriers (such as a beach umbrella). Infants over 6 months of age should be protected by a sunscreen with an SPF (sun protection factor) of 15 or higher. Older children should regularly use a sunscreen with an SPF of 15 or higher to protect against excess and repeated exposure to solar ultraviolet radiation, which can lead to skin cancer and other skin damage later in life.

Special Concerns: Zinc oxide sunscreen should be applied liberally before exposure to sunlight and reapplied every 1 to 2 hours, especially after swimming or heavy perspiration and after eating and drinking. Contact of zinc oxide with the eyes should be avoided. If skin rash or irritation develops, consult your doctor. Keep sun exposure to a minimum during peak daylight hours (10 am to 2 pm), when the sun's rays are strongest. Extra precautions should be taken around reflective surfaces such as sand, water, and concrete.

OVERDOSE
Symptoms: No specific ones have been reported.

What to Do: Not applicable. However, if someone accidentally ingests zinc oxide, immediately call a doctor, emergency medical services (EMS), or the nearest poison control center.

▼ INTERACTIONS

DRUG INTERACTIONS
Consult your doctor for specific advice if you are using any other topical medications or skin preparations.

FOOD INTERACTIONS
No known food interactions.

DISEASE INTERACTIONS
Consult your doctor for advice if you have a history of any of the following: dermatitis (skin inflammation), herpes labialis (herpes simplex of the mouth and face), lichen planus (a rare nonmalignant skin condition causing chronic itching and a distinctive skin eruption), systemic lupus erythematosus (lupus), photosensitivity (heightened sensitivity to sunlight), phytophotodermatitis (dermatitis caused by contact with certain plants followed by exposure to sunlight), polymorphous light eruption (skin lesions occurring after exposure to sunlight), or xeroderma pigmentosum (a rare genetic disorder causing extreme sensitivity to ultraviolet light, abnormal skin growths including malignancies, and serious eye problems).

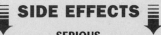

⩧ SIDE EFFECTS ⩧

SERIOUS
Acne, folliculitis (burning, pain, inflammation, and itching in hairy regions of the skin; pus in hair follicles), and skin rash may occur with zinc oxide and other physical sunscreens that block the pores. Notify your doctor if you experience such side effects.

COMMON
No common side effects have been reported.

LESS COMMON
No less-common side effects have been reported.

ZINC SULFATE OPHTHALMIC

BRAND NAMES

Clear Eyes ACR, Eye-Sed, VasoClear A, Visine Maximum Strength Allergy Relief, Zincfrin

Available in: Ophthalmic solution
Available as Generic? Yes
Drug Class: Ophthalmic astringent/analgesic

▼ USAGE INFORMATION

WHY IT'S TAKEN
For the temporary relief of discomfort and redness from minor eye irritation. It is recommended in combination with other drugs such as phenylephrine, naphazoline, and tetrahydrozoline.

HOW IT WORKS
The mineral zinc is an integral component in the proper functioning of several important enzymes involved in wound healing and the general maintenance and proper hydration of certain body tissues. Zinc sulfate ophthalmic solution has a mild astringent effect (that is, it causes tissues to contract when applied topically), which can help to shrink the tiny blood vessels in the whites of the eye (sclera) and so relieve redness and irritation.

▼ DOSAGE GUIDELINES

RANGE AND FREQUENCY
Instill 1 to 2 drops in the affected eye(s) up to 4 times a day.

ONSET OF EFFECT
Rapid.

DURATION OF ACTION
Up to several hours.

DIETARY ADVICE
No special restrictions.

STORAGE
Store in a tightly sealed container away from heat and direct light. Do not allow the solution to freeze.

MISSED DOSE
Instill the missed dose as soon as possible unless it is near the time for the next dose. In that case, skip the missed dose and go back to your regular schedule. Do not double the next dose.

STOPPING THE DRUG
You may stop applying this drug, or resume using it after discontinuing, as comfort dictates. No complications are to be expected.

PROLONGED USE
Eye drops containing zinc sulfate should generally not be used for self-medication for more than 3 days. If relief is not achieved in this time, or if redness and irritation persist or worsen, discontinue using it and contact your doctor or ophthalmologist right away.

▼ PRECAUTIONS

Over 60: No special problems are expected.

Driving and Hazardous Work: The use of this medication should not affect your ability to perform such tasks safely.

Alcohol: No special precautions are necessary.

Pregnancy: No problems are expected; however, if you are pregnant or plan to become pregnant and you have any concerns about the safe use of this or any other medication, consult your doctor.

Breast Feeding: Adequate studies on the use of ophthalmic zinc sulfate during breast feeding have not been done; however, no adverse consequences have been reported. Consult your doctor for specific advice.

Infants and Children: No specific information is available on children's use of this medication.

Special Concerns: Contact your ophthalmologist or general practitioner right away if you experience eye pain, changes in vision, or if eye irritation persists for more than 72 hours. To use the eye drops, first wash your hands. Tilt your head back. Gently apply pressure to the inside corner of the lower eyelid and with the index finger of the same hand, pull downward on the eyelid to make a space. Drop the medicine into this space and close your eye. Apply pressure for 1 or 2 minutes while keeping the eye closed without blinking. Then wash your hands again. To avoid contamination, make sure that the tip of the dropper does not touch your eye, finger, or any other surface.

OVERDOSE
Symptoms: No cases of overdose have been reported.

What to Do: An overdose is unlikely to occur; in case of accidental ingestion, call your doctor, emergency medical services (EMS), or the nearest poison control right away.

▼ INTERACTIONS

DRUG INTERACTIONS
No drug interactions have been reported, although phenylephrine, naphazoline, and tetrahydrozoline (other medications prescribed in combination with zinc sulfate ophthalmic solution) may adversely affect the action of certain glaucoma drops. Consult your doctor first before taking any other prescription or OTC eye medications.

FOOD INTERACTIONS
No known food interactions.

DISEASE INTERACTIONS
If you have glaucoma, do not use this medication without consulting your doctor first. It is not an over-the-counter substitute for antibiotic or anti-inflammatory drops. Consult your doctor for specific advice if you have any other eye disorders or a history of allergic reaction to any other ophthalmic preparations.

≡ SIDE EFFECTS ≡

SERIOUS
No serious side effects have been reported.

COMMON
Overuse of this drug may cause increased eye irritation and redness.

LESS COMMON
No less-common side effects have been reported.

ZINC SULFATE SYSTEMIC

Available in: Capsules, tablets, extended-release tablets
Available as Generic? Yes
Drug Class: Dietary supplement

▼ USAGE INFORMATION

WHY IT'S TAKEN
To prevent or treat zinc deficiency. Zinc deficiency does not occur in healthy people who eat a proper, balanced diet. Conditions associated with zinc deficiency include alcoholism, eating disorders, and intestinal problems that result from malabsorption.

HOW IT WORKS
Zinc is essential to numerous physiological processes, including the function of many enzymes in the body. Deficiency may lead to poor night vision, slow healing of wounds, poor sexual development and function in males, poor appetite (perhaps owing to a decrease in the sense of taste and smell), a reduced ability to ward off infections, diarrhea, dermatitis, and, in children, retarded growth.

▼ DOSAGE GUIDELINES

RANGE AND FREQUENCY
Recommended daily allowances are as follows: 5 to 10 mg a day for children from birth to age 3; 10 mg a day for children ages 4 to 10; 15 mg a day for adolescent and adult males; 12 mg a day for adolescent and adult females; 15 mg a day for pregnant women; and 16 to 19 mg a day for women who are breast feeding .

ONSET OF EFFECT
Unknown.

DURATION OF ACTION
Unknown.

DIETARY ADVICE
Most effective if taken 1 hour before or 2 hours after meals. It can be taken with food if stomach upset occurs.

STORAGE
Store in a tightly sealed container away from moisture, heat, and direct light.

MISSED DOSE
No cause for concern.

STOPPING THE DRUG
If you are taking zinc sulfate on your doctor's advice, speak to him or her before stopping.

PROLONGED USE
You should see your doctor regularly for tests and examinations if you take zinc sulfate for a prolonged period.

▼ PRECAUTIONS

Over 60: Zinc deficiency is more likely to occur in older persons; no special problems are expected from zinc supplementation.

Driving and Hazardous Work: The use of zinc sulfate should not impair your ability to perform such tasks safely.

Alcohol: Excessive alcohol intake can increase the likelihood of zinc deficiency.

Pregnancy: There are no known problems with recommended doses, but taking large amounts of zinc during pregnancy may be harmful to the fetus.

Breast Feeding: No problems have been reported with recommended doses.

Infants and Children: Problems have not been reported in infants and children receiving the recommended daily intake of zinc sulfate.

Special Concerns: Injectable zinc sulfate should be given under the supervision of a health care professional. Zinc is found in peas, beans, seafood such as oysters and herring, and in lean red meats. It is also found in whole grains, but consuming large amounts of whole grains can decrease the amount of zinc absorbed from the intestine. Be aware that food stored in uncoated tin cans may have less zinc available for absorption by the body.

OVERDOSE
Symptoms: Chest pain, vomiting, yellowish tinge to eyes or skin, dehydration, shortness of breath, restlessness, profuse sweating, dizziness.

What to Do: Call your doctor, emergency medical services (EMS), or the nearest poison control center immediately.

▼ INTERACTIONS

DRUG INTERACTIONS
Consult your doctor for specific advice if you are taking copper supplements or oral tetracyclines.

FOOD INTERACTIONS
Some foods can interfere with absorption of zinc sulfate into your body. Avoid taking zinc sulfate within 2 hours of eating bran, whole-wheat breads and cereals, and other fiber-rich foods, or foods containing phosphorus, such as milk and poultry.

DISEASE INTERACTIONS
Consult your doctor if you have a copper deficiency or any other medical condition. Zinc supplements make a copper deficiency worse.

≡ SIDE EFFECTS ≡

SERIOUS
Side effects are rare and occur only with large doses. Zinc itself may cause indigestion, heartburn, and nausea from irritation of the stomach. By interfering with the absorption of copper, zinc may interfere with the production of white and red blood cells, leading to infections, sores, or ulcers in the mouth or throat, and weakness due to anemia. Call your doctor if such symptoms occur.

COMMON
No common side effects have been reported.

LESS COMMON
No less-common side effects have been reported.

GLOSSARY OF DRUG TERMS

active ingredient: The chemical component in a drug preparation that exerts the desired therapeutic effects. The active ingredient is commonly what we think of as the "drug."

adverse reaction: A harmful and unintended response to a drug.

allergic drug reaction: An exaggerated immune response to a drug, which can result in hives, itching, or, in serious cases, life-threatening shock and breathing difficulties.

analgesic: An agent that relieves pain. Examples include *nonsteroidal anti-inflammatory drugs* (which have properties in addition to pain relief), and miscellaneous pain-relievers, such as capsaicin and acetaminophen.

anaphylaxis: An acute allergic reaction to a drug or venom, as from a bee sting, that may be marked by swollen airways and severe breathing difficulty.

anesthetic: A drug that eliminates the sensation of pain.

antacid: A drug that counteracts or neutralizes stomach acids. Antacids are used to relieve indigestion, heartburn, peptic ulcers, and various other gastrointestinal disorders.

antibacterial: A drug used specifically to combat bacterial infections, as opposed to infections caused by other microorganisms, such as fungi and viruses. Also commonly referred to as an antibiotic.

antibody: A protein produced by the immune system that normally acts to neutralize or eliminate foreign substances in the body. A *drug allergy* is associated with an overactive response of an antibody to a particular drug.

anticoagulant: A drug that blocks the activity of certain blood clotting factors that promote the formation of fibrin, a protein essential in the formation of blood clots.

antidiabetic agent: A drug used to treat diabetes.

antidiarrheal agent: A drug that relieves diarrhea.

antiemetic: A drug used to stop or prevent vomiting.

antifungal: A drug that combats fungal infections, such as athlete's foot or nail fungus.

antihistamine: A drug that blocks the actions of *histamine*. Such drugs relieve allergies, cold symptoms, hay fever, hives, rashes, itching, and motion sickness.

anti-inflammatory: A drug used to reduce the swelling, redness, or pain caused by inflammation, an immune reaction to injury that can occur either inside the body or on a localized external area.

antimicrobial agent: A general term for a drug used to treat infections due to microorganisms, such as bacteria, fungi, and viruses.

antipruritic: A drug that is used to relieve itching.

antipyretic: A drug used to reduce the level of a fever (an elevated body temperature).

antireflux agent: A drug that alleviates gastroesophageal reflux (heartburn).

antiseptic: A drug or other substance that arrests the growth and action of bacteria and other microorganisms.

antitussive: A cough suppressant.

antiviral: A drug used to combat infections caused by viruses, such as influenza or AIDS.

bioavailability: A scientific term for the degree and rate at which a substance, such as a drug, is absorbed into the body and available to exert therapeutic effects.

bioequivalent: A scientific term for drugs that have equivalent chemical properties, so that equal amounts of each drug are delivered to the body in a similar time frame.

brand name: The name chosen by a drug manufacturer to market a drug. Advil, for example, is the brand name for the pain reliever with the *generic name* ibuprofen.

contraceptive: A drug or device used to prevent pregnancy.

contraindication: A disease or condition that either precludes the use of a certain drug or means that the drug should be used with special caution.

decongestant: A drug that relieves nasal or sinus congestion due to colds or allergies.

desensitization: A medical treatment for a drug allergy that aims to lessen sensitivity and improve tolerance to the drug by administering, over time, a series of gradually increased doses.

divided doses: Individual doses of a drug given at intervals spaced throughout the day, rather than as a single dose.

drug allergy: An allergic reaction to a specific drug or to a drug component. Responses can range from mild (for example, a skin rash) to severe (difficulty breathing, and other signs of *anaphylaxis*).

drug interaction: Reciprocal activity or influence between two or more drugs that may alter the effects of one or all of the drugs involved. Drug interactions vary widely. They may increase—or decrease—the amount of active drug, the effectiveness of a drug, and the likelihood of adverse side effects. Responses to an interaction range from mild to life-threatening.

drug rash: A skin rash resulting from an allergic reaction to a particular medication, usually appearing during the first few days after taking it.

emollient: A drug preparation or other substance that soothes and softens the skin, lips, or mucous membranes.

expectorant: A type of medication commonly used in cough preparations that promotes the discharge and expulsion of mucus or phlegm from the throat and airways.

food interactions: An action between a specific food and a drug, which may influence the amount of drug available for therapeutic effects.

g or gm: An abbreviation for *gram*.

generic name: The scientific name for a drug. Generic names, as opposed to *brand names*, are nonproprietary and are recognized worldwide.

gram (g): A metric measure of weight, sometimes used in drug dosages. There are about 454 grams in a pound.

histamine: A compound produced by cells in the body. Histamine aids digestion by triggering stomach acid secretion. It also plays a key role in allergic reactions, causing inflammation, hives, itching, and constriction of the airways.

hypersensitivity: An exaggerated response to a drug, or a drug-related allergic reaction.

hypoglycemic agent: A drug that lowers blood sugar levels, commonly used in the treatment of diabetes.

immunization: Stimulation of the immune system to produce antibodies against a specific disease, thereby conferring protection against it. The term is sometimes used interchangeably with vaccination.

implant: A capsule implanted under the skin that slowly releases a drug into the body for an extended period.

inactive ingredient: A substance, such as a coloring, flavoring, binder, gelatin capsule coating, or preservative, that does not have any therapeutic effects but that is combined with an active drug compound during the manufacturing process to make a drug.

indication: The disorder, condition, disease, or symptom for which a drug is prescribed or approved for use by the Food and Drug Administration.

kilogram (kg): A metric unit of weight equal to about 2.2 pounds.

laxative: One of a group of drugs that relieves constipation by adding bulk to fecal matter, softening the stools, lubricating the gastrointestinal tract, or increasing intestinal tract motility.

mcg: An abbreviation for *microgram*.

mEq: An abbreviation for *milliequivalent*.

mg: An abbreviation for *milligram*.

microgram (mcg): A metric measure of weight, equal to one-millionth of a *gram*, that is used in drug dosages.

milliequivalent (mEq): A chemical unit of measure that is sometimes used to indicate dosages of vitamins and some drugs.

milligram (mg): A metric measure of weight, equal to one-thousandth of a *gram*, that is used in drug dosages.

milliliter (mL): A metric measure of volume, equal to one-thousandth of a liter, that is commonly used in liquid medication dosing.

mineral: An inorganic substance, found in the earth's crust, that plays a crucial role in the human body for enzyme synthesis, regulation of heart rhythm, bone formation, digestion, and other metabolic processes.

mL: An abbreviation for *milliliter*.

mucolytic: A type of drug that is used in the treatment of coughs and other types of upper respiratory congestion to thin mucus secretions.

nonsteroidal anti-inflammatory drug (NSAID): A type of drug that reduces pain and inflammation in such conditions as arthritis by blocking the production of specialized hormone-like chemicals called prostaglandins.

ophthalmic: A drug that has been formulated for administration into or around the eye.

otic: A drug that has been formulated for administration into the ear or onto the surface of the ear.

overdose: Excessive accumulation of a drug in the body, resulting in toxic levels that can be dangerous.

photosensitivity: An adverse *side effect* of certain medications marked by a decreased tolerance to the sun's ultraviolet rays, resulting in a tendency for exposed skin to sunburn easily.

side effect: A secondary, and often adverse, effect of a drug. Side effects are known and predictable responses to a specific drug, though usually only a small minority of patients taking the drug will be affected by them.

stool softener: A type of *laxative* that bulks up and softens fecal matter, easing the passage of stools.

systemic: Affecting the body in general, as opposed to a limited local area. Drugs taken orally or injected intravenously, for example, are sometimes called systemic medications, since they are distributed throughout the body by the bloodstream.

ACKNOWLEDGMENTS

▼

MEDICAL CONSULTANTS

*Chief of Medical
Advisory Board*
Simeon Margolis, M.D., Ph.D.
*Professor of Medicine and
Biological Chemistry
Johns Hopkins
School of Medicine*

Franklin Adkinson, M.D.
Asthma and Allergy Medicine

Frank Anania, M.D.
*Gastroenterology and
Hepatology*

Lawrence Appel, M.D.
Internal Medicine

Paul Auwaerter, M.D.
*Internal Medicine and
Infectious Disease*

William Bell, M.D.
Hematology

Ivan Borrello, M.D.
Oncology

Steven Brant, M.D.
Gastroenterology

Richard Chaisson, M.D.
Infectious Disease

Lawrence Cheskin, M.D.
Gastroenterology and Nutrition

Bernard Cohen, M.D.
Dermatology

David Cromwell, M.D.
Gastroenterology

E. Claire Dees, M.D.
Oncology

Phillip Dennis, M.D.
Oncology

Adrian Dobs, M.D.
Endocrinology

Christopher Earley, M.D.
Neurology

David Essayan, M.D.
Allergy and Immunology

John Flynn, M.D.
*Internal Medicine and
Rheumatology*

Joel Gallant, M.D.
Infectious Disease (HIV/AIDS)

Mary Lawrence Harris, M.D.
Gastroenterology

Bradley Hinz, M.D.
Ophthalmology

Thomas Inglesby, M.D.
*Internal Medicine and
Infectious Disease*

Suzanne Jan de Beur, M.D.
Endocrinology

Christopher Karp, M.D.
Parasitology

Beth Kirkpatrick, M.D.
Infectious Disease

Susan Koch, M.D.
Dermatology

Alan Krasner, M.D.
Endocrinology

Julie Krop, M.D.
Endocrinology and Metabolism

Ralph Kuncl, M.D.
Neurology

John Lawrence, M.D.
Cardiovascular Medicine

Linda Lee, M.D.
Gastroenterology

Ronald Lesser, M.D.
Neurology

John Lipsey, M.D.
Psychiatry

Dan Martin, M.D.
*Internal Medicine and
Rheumatology*

William Moss, M.D.
Immunology

Patrick Murphy, M.D.
Infectious Disease

Philip Norman, M.D.
Allergy and Immunology

Steve O'Connell, M.D.
Ophthalmology

Paul O'Donnell, M.D.
Oncology

Peter Pak, M.D.
Cardiology

Marco Pappagallo, M.D.
*Neurology (Chronic Pain
Management)*

Wendy Post, M.D.
Cardiovascular Medicine

Charles Pound, M.D.
Urology

Thomas Preziosi, M.D.
Neurology

Peter Rabins, M.D.
Neuropsychiatry

Stuart Ray, M.D.
*Internal Medicine and
Infectious Disease*

Jon Resar, M.D.
Cardiovascular Medicine

Beryl Rosenstein, M.D.
Pulmonary Medicine

Walter Royal, M.D.
Neurology and Virology

Christopher Saudek, M.D.
Endocrinology and Metabolism

Eduardo Sotomayor, M.D.
Oncology

Jerry Spivak, M.D.
Hematology

Timothy Sterling, M.D.
Infectious Disease

Francisco Tausk, M.D.
Dermatology

Peter Terry, M.D.
Asthma and Allergy Medicine

Chloe Thio, M.D.
Infectious Disease

Jason Thompson, M.D.
Nephrology

Thomas Traill, M.D.
Cardiovascular Medicine

Glenn Treisman, M.D.
Psychiatry

John Ulatowski, M.D.
Neurology

Edward Wallach, M.D.
Obstetrics and Gynecology

Gary Wand, M.D.
Endocrinology

James Weiss, M.D.
Cardiovascular Medicine

James Weisz, M.D.
Ophthalmology

Elizabeth Whitmore, M.D.
Dermatology

INDEX

▼

GENERIC drug names appear in capital letters.

GENERIC drug names appear in capital letters.

GENERIC drug names appear in capital letters.